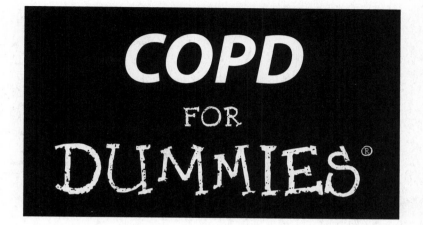

COPD FOR DUMMIES®

by Kevin Felner, MD, and Meg Schneider

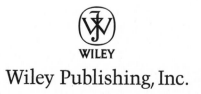

WILEY

Wiley Publishing, Inc.

COPD For Dummies®

Published by
Wiley Publishing, Inc.
111 River St.
Hoboken, NJ 07030-5774
www.wiley.com

Copyright © 2008 by Wiley Publishing, Inc., Indianapolis, Indiana

Published simultaneously in Canada

For general information on our other products and services, please contact our Customer Care Department within the U.S. at 800-762-2974, outside the U.S. at 317-572-3993, or fax 317-572-4002.

For technical support, please visit www.wiley.com/techsupport.

Wiley also publishes its books in a variety of electronic formats. Some content that appears in print may not be available in electronic books.

Library of Congress Control Number: 2008924951

ISBN: 978-0-470-24757-0

Manufactured in the United States of America

10 9 8 7 6 5 4 3 2 1

WILEY

About the Authors

Kevin Felner, MD: Kevin Felner, MD, an assistant professor at New York University School of Medicine in New York City, is an expert in pulmonary and critical care medicine. He served a three-year fellowship at New York University Medical Center in pulmonary/critical care medicine and has taught medical students in his specialty (Department of Internal Medicine/ Division of Pulmonary and Critical Care) since 2004. He has earned three Teacher of the Year awards during his tenure at NYU, including being named best teacher of the Division of Pulmonary and Critical Care in 2005.

Before joining the NYU teaching staff, he taught at UT Southwestern Medical School and Mount Sinai Medical School, where he participated in pilot programs introducing first- and second-year medical students to effective patient interaction.

His research on lung and respiratory illnesses has been presented to the American Thoracic Society and published in journals such as the *International Journal of Surgical Pathology*.

Kevin earned his undergraduate and medical degrees from Emory University in Atlanta, where he received, among other honors, the Mrs. L. V. (Ola) Hammack Memorial Scholarship.

Kevin lives in New York City with his wife, Galit, and their son, Liam.

Meg Schneider: Meg Schneider is an award-winning writer with more than two decades of experience in television, radio, and print journalism and public relations. Meg has authored or coauthored several books, including *The Birth Order Effect for Couples* (Fair Winds Press) and *The Good-For-You Marriage* (Adams Media). Her other book credits include two books for writers and one on casino gambling.

Meg's journalism honors include awards from the Iowa Associated Press Managing Editors, Women in Communications, the Maryland-Delaware-D.C. Press Association, Gannett, the New York State Associated Press, and the William Randolph Hearst Foundation.

A native of Iowa, Meg now lives in upstate New York.

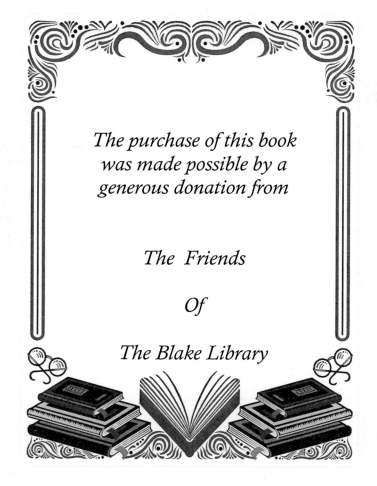

The purchase of this book was made possible by a generous donation from

The Friends

Of

The Blake Library

Dedication

Kevin dedicates this book to his wife, Galit, and son, Liam, whose love and support are the foundation of all he does and aspires to.

Meg dedicates this book to Bob and Helen Abel, for whose friendship and love she is grateful beyond words.

Authors' Acknowledgments

The tricky thing about acknowledgements is that you're always in danger of inadvertently forgetting to mention someone who will be mortally offended at the omission. On the other hand, if, in an attempt to include everyone, you dither on about the inspiration you received from Tom This, the encouragement of Dick That, and the patience of Harry the Other, not to mention the late-night coffee-and-ice-cream-sessions with Jane So-and-So and the eternal friendship of Sally Such-and-Such, your readers get restless. "Who *are* these people?" they fume to themselves, anxiously skimming the pages to see where the acknowledgements section finally ends. "Get on with it already!"

So. In the interests of brevity (and at the risk of being written out of someone's will), the authors offer their thanks to the following people:

The folks at Wiley, for recognizing the importance of arming readers with information about COPD and for supporting this book to fill that need.

Our editors, Tracy Boggier and Elizabeth Kuball, for their vision, support, patience, and dedication.

Our agent, Barb Doyen, for bringing us together on this project and acting as business partner, cheerleader, coach, and friend.

Nick Pastis, for making sure we didn't go off the rails.

Galit and Liam Felner, for all their patience, love, and understanding.

Mark Dixon, for hanging in there through all the loopiness.

And, finally, all those we should have included by name but didn't, for their forbearance and (we hope) forgiveness.

Publisher's Acknowledgments

We're proud of this book; please send us your comments through our Dummies online registration form located at www.dummies.com/register/.

Some of the people who helped bring this book to market include the following:

Acquisitions, Editorial, and Media Development

Project Editor: Elizabeth Kuball

Acquisitions Editor: Tracy Boggier

Copy Editor: Elizabeth Kuball

Editorial Program Coordinator: Erin Calligan Mooney

Technical Editor: Nicholas J. Pastis, Jr., MD

Senior Editorial Manager: Jennifer Ehrlich

Editorial Supervisor and Reprint Editor: Carmen Krikorian

Editorial Assistants: Joe Niesen, David Lutton

Art Coordinator: Alicia B. South

Cover Photo: 3DClinic

Cartoons: Rich Tennant (www.the5thwave.com)

Composition Services

Project Coordinator: Katie Key

Layout and Graphics: Reuben W. Davis, Alissa D. Ellet, Stephanie D. Jumper, Christine Williams

Special Art: Kathryn Born

Proofreaders: Laura Albert, Broccoli Information Management

Indexer: Broccoli Information Management

Publishing and Editorial for Consumer Dummies

    Diane Graves Steele, Vice President and Publisher, Consumer Dummies

    Joyce Pepple, Acquisitions Director, Consumer Dummies

    Kristin A. Cocks, Product Development Director, Consumer Dummies

    Michael Spring, Vice President and Publisher, Travel

    Kelly Regan, Editorial Director, Travel

Publishing for Technology Dummies

    Andy Cummings, Vice President and Publisher, Dummies Technology/General User

Composition Services

    Gerry Fahey, Vice President of Production Services

    Debbie Stailey, Director of Composition Services

Contents at a Glance

Table of Contents

Introduction

Chronic obstructive pulmonary disease (COPD) — involving chronic bronchitis, emphysema, or both — is the fourth leading cause of death and the second leading cause of disability in the United States. Twelve million Americans have been diagnosed with COPD, and experts believe another 12 million suffer from COPD but don't know it.

COPD is a progressive disease, meaning it develops and gets worse over time. You don't just wake up one morning and realize you have COPD. Instead, you find that activities that used to be easy for you are harder now. You may become breathless walking upstairs, or you may have trouble carrying groceries into the house. You may not have the energy to eat at night, and this may lead to weight loss and a feeling of overall weakness. Even when you're sitting quietly, you may feel like you can't catch your breath.

And you may attribute all these symptoms to age, because COPD usually doesn't begin to make itself noticed until you're in your 40s, 50s, or 60s.

Part of the reason COPD is so severely under-diagnosed is that many physicians mistake its symptoms for other illnesses, particularly asthma. But effective treatments for asthma and COPD differ, and if you're being treated for asthma when you really suffer from COPD, chances are, your symptoms won't improve much.

And that leads us to another common misconception about COPD: that it cannot be treated. True, after damage is done to your lungs by smoking or other factors, that damage can't be reversed. But when it is properly diagnosed, COPD can be treated effectively, and with the proper treatment, you don't have to let COPD keep you from doing the things you enjoy.

About This Book

Our objective in writing this book is twofold. First, we want you to understand COPD — its causes and effects and why it makes you feel the way you do. We show you how your lungs work and how COPD interferes with your lung function. We talk about how impaired breathing affects the rest of your body. We discuss the differences between COPD and other lung diseases like asthma and tuberculosis. And we put all this technical medical stuff in plain, easy-to-understand language, so you'll know what your doctor is talking about when he tosses off terms like *alveoli* and *forced expiratory volume.*

Second, we want you to know what you can do about COPD. Too often, people who are diagnosed with this disease feel powerless to improve their quality of life. But with the proper care and attention to your condition and your overall health, you can help yourself get the most out of living with COPD. Part of what you can do about it involves medications prescribed by your doctor — but that's only part of it. Nutrition and exercise play big roles in treating COPD and slowing its progress, and those two areas are up to you. We give you the information you need to make wise choices when it comes to eating and physical activity. Finally, we show you ways you can adapt to your condition without letting it dictate your life. Changes in your daily routine and the way certain areas of your home are organized can make life much easier for you, preserving your sense of independence and ability to enjoy life.

Conventions Used in This Book

For the sake of consistency and readability, we use the following conventions throughout the text:

- ✔ Medical and technical terms are in *italics,* and plain-English explanations of their meanings are nearby in the text, often in parentheses.

- ✔ When we give you steps to follow in a particular order, we put the action part of each step in **bold.**

- ✔ E-mail addresses and Web addresses are in `monofont`. ***Note:*** When this book was printed, some Web addresses may have needed to break across two lines of text. If that happened, rest assured that we haven't put in any extra characters (such as hyphens) to indicate the break. So, when using one of these Web addresses, just type in exactly what you see in this book, pretending as though the line break doesn't exist.

What You're Not to Read

This book is structured so that you can find the specific information you're looking for without wading through a bunch of stuff you don't care about. You don't have to read the chapters in any particular order; you don't even have to read all of them if you don't want to.

Occasionally, you'll see sidebars — shaded boxes of text that go into detail on a particular topic. You don't have to read these if you're not interested; skipping them won't hamper you in understanding the rest of the text. You also can skip any information next to the Technical Stuff icon. Again, this information is presented for the intensely curious reader, but you won't be missing anything crucial if you ignore it.

Foolish Assumptions

In putting together the information in this book, we've made some assumptions about you, the reader. We assume that you:

- ✔ Have been diagnosed with COPD, suspect you may have COPD, or have a loved one who has COPD.
- ✔ Want to understand how your lungs work and how your lung function affects the rest of your body.
- ✔ Want information about what a COPD diagnosis means.
- ✔ Want to understand your treatment options.
- ✔ Want to know how you can manage COPD effectively with medication and lifestyle choices.
- ✔ Want tips on how to make the lifestyle choices that will help you manage your COPD.
- ✔ Want a convenient, comprehensive, and easy-to-understand resource that covers all this information without making you feel like a dummy.

How This Book Is Organized

We split this book into five parts to make it easier for you to find the information you're looking for. Here's how it's organized.

Part 1: Every Breath You Take: The Who, What, and Why of COPD

This part covers the mechanics of COPD. We talk about the two lung diseases that comprise COPD — chronic bronchitis and emphysema — as well as other lung ailments that COPD can be mistaken for. We also show you how your lungs normally work and how COPD prevents them from working properly. And we discuss various risk factors for COPD, starting with the number-one risk, smoking, and going right through other risks like exposure to airborne contaminants and a rare but serious genetic condition that almost inevitably leads to COPD.

Part II: Catching Your Breath: Treating COPD

In these chapters, we walk you through the process of diagnosing and treating COPD. We tell you what kinds of tests your doctor may order and how to help determine the severity of your condition. Because COPD patients often suffer from depression, especially when they're first diagnosed, we talk about the common emotional reactions to a COPD diagnosis and give you tips on finding support and coping with your own emotional response.

Because COPD affects virtually every aspect of your life, we show you how to build a health-care team that can address every facet, from medical treatment to diet to exercises designed to help you breathe better. We also discuss the importance of setting goals for your treatment and how to assess your progress.

This part also covers the various medications used to treat COPD symptoms, including why they help, how to use them, and what side effects you may experience from each. We also cover surgical and alternative treatment options and discuss when these options make sense, as well as factors you and your doctor need to consider before using them.

Part III: In the Next Breath: Managing Your Overall Health

Getting the right medications for the problems in your lungs is only part of living with COPD. Quitting smoking, getting appropriate exercise, and making sure you eat a balanced diet that also provides you with enough calories are all critical components of treating your COPD. We show you how these things affect your condition (and how COPD affects these things) and provide information and tips for managing your general health as well as your COPD.

Part IV: Breathing Easier: Living with COPD

COPD robs you of energy. Simple tasks like running the vacuum, taking a stroll, even bathing and getting dressed can seem monumental when you have COPD. In this part, we provide tips for making your daily routine less tiring, showing you how to gauge your energy levels, choose clothing that's more comfortable and meals that are more appetizing, and reorganize your home and daily routine to make life with COPD easier.

This part also provides essential information on preparing for emergencies. Here you find the signs that mean you need medical help immediately.

If you have a loved one with COPD, this part also provides a quick primer to understanding the effects of COPD. This is where you'll find information on what you need to know about your loved one's condition and medications, tips on how you can help your loved one manage the disease, and a guide to help you identify danger signs.

Part V: The Part of Tens

A favorite feature of *For Dummies* books, the Part of Tens gives you quick, easily digestible nuggets of information. Here we present our top-ten lists for living with and understanding COPD, including ten things to avoid when you have COPD and ten common myths about the disease. We also give you ten strategies for coping with COPD on a daily basis, and ten health factors that affect COPD (or vice versa).

Glossary

Although we explain any technical terms in the text, sometimes it's easier to look up an unfamiliar word in a glossary format, rather than having to hunt through the text for the definition. This glossary is intended to be a handy and reasonably thorough guide to understanding what your doctor is talking about.

Icons Used in This Book

Throughout the book, you'll find little icons in the margins that alert you to specific kinds of information. Here's what each of the icons means:

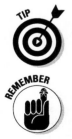

This is practical information that you can use right away to make a specific task easier.

This icon indicates information that you may want to file away for future reference.

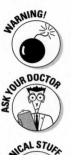

This little bomb tips you off to potential problems or dangers you should be aware of.

Because everyone's medical needs are different, we use this icon to remind you when you should consult your physician before taking a specific course of action.

When we get into technical medical stuff, we alert you with this icon so you can skip it if you want.

Where to Go from Here

The beauty of Dummies books is that you can use them in whatever way works best for you. You can start with Chapter 1 and work your way to the last page, or you can peruse the table of contents, decide which area seems most inter-esting or useful to you at the moment, and start your reading there. Either way, our goal is that you find and take away a better understanding of COPD.

Still not sure where to start? Here are our recommendations:

- ✔ If you've just been diagnosed with COPD, head to Chapter 7 for informa-tion on treatment goals. Chapter 5 can help you deal with how you feel about the diagnosis, and Chapters 8 and 9 cover various medical treatments.

- ✔ If you're trying to manage your COPD better, go to Chapter 11 for nutrition information and Chapter 12 for information on exercising with COPD.

- ✔ If a loved one has COPD, start with Chapter 17 to find out what you can do to help. You also can use the information in Chapters 14 and 15 to help your loved one remain independent.

Part I
Every Breath You Take: The Who, What, and Why of COPD

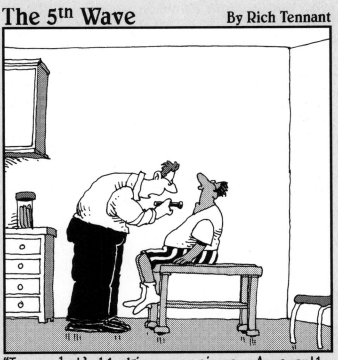

"I see what's blocking your airway. Apparently, someone said something at some point that just stuck in your craw."

In this part . . .

COPD is often misdiagnosed as asthma or another lung ailment. Because it's a progressive disease, people often don't notice or seek medical treatment for their symptoms until the damage is fairly well advanced. In this part, we explain the differences between COPD and other lung diseases and identify common ways in which early-stage COPD can make its presence felt.

We also take you inside your body's respiratory system to show you how it functions when it's healthy and when it's not, and we look at factors that influence how well your lungs function. Then we give you detailed information about the risk factors for COPD — from smoking to gender to individual medical history — so you can assess how many of these factors apply to you.

Chapter 1

Understanding COPD

. . . .

. . . .

Chronic obstructive pulmonary disease, or COPD, is the fourth leading cause of death in the United States and the second leading cause of disability. The costs associated with COPD are enormous — more than $37 billion a year, including $20 billion a year just in direct healthcare costs. Some 12 million American adults have been diagnosed with COPD, and another 12 million may have it but don't know it.

How can there be so many undiagnosed cases of a life-threatening illness? For the same reason that many diabetics and people with high blood pressure go undiagnosed: The symptoms, especially early on, are so vague that they're easy to ignore. And when COPD symptoms do appear, they can be mistaken for other conditions, like asthma.

In fact, until fairly recently, most people outside the health profession had never heard of COPD, and those who had heard of it very often dismissed it as a "smoker's disease." Smoking is the number-one risk factor for COPD, but it is by no means the only one. Long-term exposure to dust, chemical fumes, secondhand smoke, and other pollutants can lead to COPD, and there's even a genetic condition that, though rare, can cause the disease.

COPD also was long considered a man's disease. But since 2003, more women than men have died every year from COPD. Many experts attribute this shift to the fact that, while smoking rates among men have dropped over the past two or three decades, the smoking rates for women have crept upward. Women also seem to suffer more than men from many of the health-sapping effects of COPD, so it tends to progress faster in women than it does in men.

That's the insidious thing about COPD: It's a progressive disease. New treatments and better understanding have improved management of its symptoms, but there is no cure, and the average life expectancy after diagnosis is about five years, depending on the severity of the COPD and other health factors.

Faced with these sobering facts, many people feel overwhelmed, even discouraged or depressed, when they first learn they have COPD. But you aren't completely powerless. There are all kinds of steps you can take to manage your COPD symptoms and improve your quality of life. The first step is understanding COPD and how it affects your body.

What COPD Is and Isn't

COPD is an umbrella term covering any long-term, irreversible damage to the lungs that interferes with breathing, specifically with getting air out of the lungs.

If you break the term down into its four parts, here's what *chronic obstructive pulmonary disease* means:

- *Chronic* means "always present" (as opposed to *acute,* which refers to a short-term condition that disappears after treatment).
- *Obstructive* means "blocking."
- *Pulmonary* refers to the lungs, including the airways and tissues that allow your body to pull in oxygen and push out carbon dioxide and other gases.
- *Disease* is a condition that harms a specific bodily function and/or your overall health.

So *chronic obstructive pulmonary disease* is a condition in which you have trouble getting air out of your lungs because your airways are continually blocked.

Not being able to get air out is a problem because, when that air is trapped in your lungs, you can't inhale enough air to supply your body with oxygen. (Chapter 2 describes the gas exchange process in detail.) Your body senses that you aren't getting enough oxygen and sends signals telling you to breathe faster to correct the problem. This process is what makes you feel like you can't catch your breath.

Smoking just adds to the problem. Smoking increases mucous production in your lungs and paralyzes the *cilia* — the little "brooms" whose job it is to sweep mucus and particles up your airways so they can be coughed out. Too much mucus clogs the gas-exchange function of your air sacs, so you feel short of breath.

When you can't cough out mucus and particles, you have a higher risk of developing lung infections like pneumonia — a serious problem for COPD patients.

Coughing is one of your respiratory system's most important defense mechanisms. But smoking can interfere with your ability to cough effectively. You may not be able to cough out as much air, and you may not be able to put enough force behind your cough to expel mucus and irritants. The smoker's hack, though more frequent than a nonsmoker's cough, isn't nearly as effective.

What COPD is: The deadly combo

In the vast majority of patients, at least in the United States, COPD refers to a combination of chronic bronchitis and emphysema. (Other countries have higher incidences of other lung diseases that can fall under the definition of COPD.) Most COPD patients have both conditions, although one may be more advanced than the other.

Chronic bronchitis

Bronchitis is a condition in which the airways in your lungs are inflamed, making them narrower. Inflammation is usually a response to an irritant, like cigarette smoke, dust, or pollen. When your airways are irritated, they create more mucus in an effort to rid your lungs of the irritants. But this.extra mucus, combined with the narrowing of the airways themselves, can end up blocking your airways. Air then gets trapped in your lungs, and you feel short of breath.

In chronic bronchitis, your airways become scarred and the partial blockage is permanent. Extra mucus is produced all the time, which can make you feel congested and prompt continual coughing. You become more susceptible to respiratory infections because the extra mucus in your airways provides an admirable breeding ground for bacteria and viruses. Figure 1-1 shows how chronic bronchitis affects your airways.

Chronic bronchitis develops over several years. It can affect people of any age, but it is most common in smokers who are in their 40s or older. About 9 million Americans have been diagnosed with chronic bronchitis; two-thirds of them are female.

Symptoms include chronic coughing and throat clearing, increased mucus, and shortness of breath. To meet the clinical definition of chronic bronchitis, you must cough up mucus most days for at least three months of the year for two consecutive years.

Many people ignore their chronic bronchitis symptoms because they mistakenly believe it isn't serious. The earlier you see your doctor, the better your chances of preventing serious damage to your lungs.

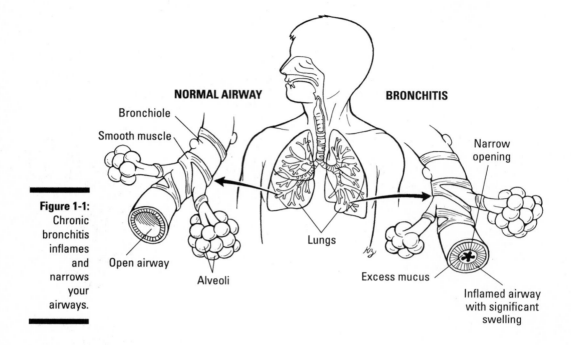

NORMAL AIRWAY

Bronchiole

Smooth muscle

BRONCHITIS

Narrow opening

Figure 1-1:
Chronic bronchitis inflames and narrows your airways.

Open airway

Lungs

Alveoli

Excess mucus

Inflamed airway with significant swelling

Emphysema

Chronic bronchitis affects your airways, the tubes that branch out into your lungs. Emphysema affects the tiny air sacs at the ends of your airways. This is where the oxygen in the air you inhale is exchanged for carbon dioxide and other waste material in your blood. To facilitate this exchange, the walls of your air sacs naturally are quite thin and fragile. In emphysema, the walls of the air sacs are stretched, distended, and eventually destroyed, leaving permanent holes in your lungs. The fewer air sacs there are, the more difficult the *gas exchange* — trading oxygen from inhaled air for carbon dioxide in your blood — becomes, and this can contribute to you feeling short of breath. Figure 1-2 shows how emphysema affects your lungs.

Emphysema takes time to develop; nine out of ten people diagnosed with it are 45 or older. In the past, men have been slightly more likely than women to be diagnosed with emphysema, but the balance is beginning to shift as smoking rates for women rise while those for men decline.

Early symptoms of emphysema are vague and often attributed to age rather than to any lung problem. Most people figure their cough is from smoking and their shortness of breath is from the infamous "middle-age spread," so they don't consider it worth mentioning to their doctors. By the time symptoms begin to cause concern — like feeling short of breath even while sitting or lying down — emphysema has caused quite a bit of damage.

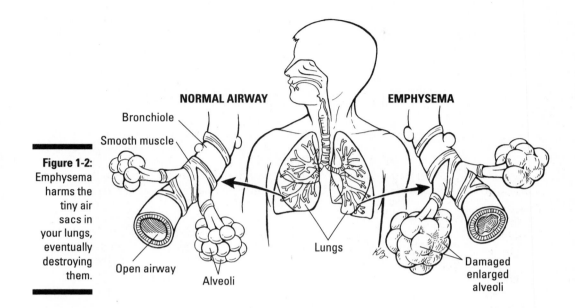

Emphysema also robs your lungs of their elasticity, which can cause smaller airways to collapse, thus trapping more air in the lower lungs. This can make it difficult to bring in new air for gas exchanges, which worsens the function of your respiratory muscles, which makes you work harder at breathing, which makes you feel short of breath.

What COPD isn't: Other lung ailments

COPD is easily mistaken for other lung diseases because the symptoms of so many different ailments are similar. In particular, COPD is often misdiagnosed — and treated — as asthma. (See Chapter 4 for information on diagnosing COPD and ruling out other lung diseases.) And, because mild COPD can so easily be ignored or taken for an acute illness like a cold or acute bronchitis, patients often overlook the early signs of COPD.

In the following sections, we cover other lung ailments that COPD is often mistaken for.

Asthma

Asthma is similar to COPD in that it blocks the flow of air out of the lungs. But that's only true when you have an asthma attack. In between attacks, lung function is usually good. In COPD, lung function is always impaired to some extent.

Asthma patients have what doctors call *reversible airway obstruction.* COPD patients typically have irreversible or minimally reversible airway obstruction.

Medicines called *bronchodilators* open up the airways during an asthma attack and restore normal air flow. Those same medications are used to treat COPD and are effective at partially reversing the airflow obstruction. As COPD progresses, however, bronchodilators become less effective.

In some cases, people with asthma can develop permanent airway obstruction, so their lung function doesn't return to normal in between attacks. They lose the reversible quality of their obstruction to the effects of chronic inflammation. When that happens, these asthma sufferers have lung disease that is indistinguishable from COPD, so it's sometimes referred to as *asthmatic COPD.*

Asthma usually develops early in life, while COPD is rare in people under age 40. COPD is strongly linked to smoking, while asthma is not uncommon in nonsmokers. And although both conditions include the possibility of sudden attacks, asthma attacks usually are sparked by identifiable triggers like allergens and often end when the trigger is removed. In COPD, suddenly worse symptoms may take weeks to resolve.

Respiratory infections

Pneumonia, tuberculosis, and pleurisy are all acute infections — that is, short-term illnesses that go away with proper treatment. They usually produce symptoms that are rare with COPD, including fever, headaches or muscle aches, and chills. However, even though these illnesses aren't the same as COPD, people who have COPD are more susceptible to respiratory infections.

Pneumonia can occur in one or both lungs, and it can be caused by bacteria, viruses, or fungi. The organisms that cause pneumonia normally settle in the air sacs in the lower lungs, which fill with fluid and pus in reaction to the invasion. In some cases, pneumonia can cause permanent lung damage.

Tuberculosis, or TB, can look similar to COPD, but, like pneumonia, it's really a respiratory infection caused by bacteria, not a result of damage over a period of years.

Pneumonia and pulmonary TB are contagious; COPD is *not.* You can't "catch" COPD except through long-term exposure to lung-damaging substances like tobacco smoke.

Lung cancer

Smoking is a risk factor for both COPD and lung cancer, and COPD itself is a risk factor for lung cancer. But COPD is *not* cancer, and being diagnosed with COPD doesn't mean you'll automatically develop lung cancer.

How COPD Affects Your Body

COPD steals your energy, which has a cascade effect through the rest of your body. It's a gradual loss, which is why early COPD symptoms are so often ignored — if they're noticed at all. Many people with mild COPD don't have any symptoms beyond a vague tendency to get tired more quickly than they used to. But, as the disease progresses, the lack of energy becomes far more pronounced, overall physical weakness increases, and COPD sufferers find that even the smallest of tasks drains them of whatever energy they have.

Loss of energy

In people with healthy lungs, normal breathing doesn't take a lot of energy. In fact, healthy people only use energy to breathe when they inhale, to inflate the lungs; exhaling is more or less a passive activity because healthy lungs are elastic and push air out on their own when they spring back to their normal position.

With COPD, the lungs lose that elastic quality, so you have to use extra energy to force air out of your lungs. You use twice the energy just to breathe.

You also have to breathe more often when you have COPD, because the air that's trapped in your lungs reduces the volume of air you can take in with your next breath. The gas exchange is less efficient, so your body doesn't have as much oxygen to fuel itself.

COPD patients use more calories to breathe, and that leaves fewer calories to nourish the muscles. On top of that, many COPD patients find that they're too tired to prepare or eat meals, so their caloric intake drops even as their bodies use up more of the calories they do take in to do the job of breathing. This energy drain is so significant that some COPD patients may use as much as ten times more calories than healthy people.

Unfortunately, the energy drain also makes it harder for people with COPD to get the nutrition they need. The digestion process itself takes a great deal of energy, so people with COPD often don't feel like eating. Medications used to treat COPD can affect appetite, as well. And preparing food can be tiring, so when people with COPD do feel like eating, they're more likely to go for prepackaged convenience foods, which can contain sodium and other ingredients that aren't good for either their lungs or their overall health.

Loss of muscle strength

The lack of oxygen and sufficient calorie intake leads to loss of muscle mass and strength. This is why exercise is such a critical component of a comprehensive treatment plan for COPD. Aerobic exercise like walking or riding a stationary bike helps bring more oxygen into your body and tone your muscles, including the muscles involved in breathing. This kind of conditioning has been shown to reduce symptoms of being short of breath and improve overall quality of life for COPD patients, no matter how far their illness has progressed.

Exercise has other benefits of particular importance to COPD patients, too. COPD is often accompanied by heart disease or circulatory problems, and exercise can help make your heart and circulatory system stronger; exercise is known to help control blood pressure and improve the heart's ability to pump blood efficiently. A regular exercise regimen improves sleep quality, which helps you feel more energetic, and it promotes better posture, balance, and flexibility.

Exercise also is effective in counteracting many of the emotional effects of the disease. Forced inactivity can lead to a sense of isolation and depression; exercise is a proven mood brightener and self-confidence booster.

Working harder for fewer results

As COPD progresses, patients find that it takes more energy to do less. Even relatively passive activities like reaching for something on a shelf or bending over to pick up something from the floor can leave people with severe COPD feeling exhausted. So much of the body's resources are diverted to the task of breathing that, eventually, there's next to nothing left over for other activities.

The goal of virtually every COPD treatment plan is to fend off this stage of the disease for as long as possible. The right combination of medications, nutrition, exercise, and emotional and social support is far more effective in achieving this goal than any individual element can be.

How COPD Affects Your Life

The impact COPD has on your life depends on how far it has progressed and how severe your symptoms are. Many people with mild COPD find that it doesn't affect their daily routine much at all, beyond perhaps an occasional cough and a tendency to tire a little more quickly. Moderate COPD may dictate changes in routines and adjustments to both the number and intensity of activities you can engage in.

Severe COPD has the most dramatic impact on your daily life. At this stage, you may no longer have the energy to do even simple tasks like bathing and getting dressed, much less more demanding things like mowing the lawn or shopping for groceries.

Missing work

COPD is the second-leading cause of disability in the United States, behind only arthritis. Mild COPD may prompt you to take more sick days than you used to because you tire more easily. Moderate COPD can force you to change from a physically demanding job to a more sedentary one; many people with moderate COPD leave their full-time jobs in favor of part-time ones because their symptoms don't leave enough energy for a full-time job. By the time COPD reaches the severe stage, very few people are able to continue working at all; they just don't have enough energy to do it.

Aside from issues of fatigue, there are risks in continuing to work while you have COPD. Your immune system isn't as strong, so you're more susceptible to whatever bug may be making the rounds at your workplace. If your job involves a lot of physical exertion or exposure to dust, fumes, or other irritants, continuing to work may do more harm to your health. And overexertion can lead to sudden worsening of your symptoms, which can become life-threatening episodes.

Skipping social activities

The continual fatigue associated with COPD prompts most patients to cut back on their social and recreational activities — sometimes without even realizing how much they've cut back. One of the challenges of living with COPD is figuring out how to use limited stores of energy; without forethought and planning, many COPD patients find themselves dropping out of the things they used to find most enjoyable in their lives.

Unfortunately, social isolation can make COPD — and any other chronic illness — even worse, because it's a key factor in depression. Recent research has shown that depression actually is harder on your general health than many chronic illnesses like diabetes and arthritis, and when depression accompanies a chronic illness, the illness itself is worse.

Doing less at home

Eventually, COPD interferes with your ability to do any activities, even mundane household chores. You can't carry as much as you used to, and pushing the vacuum across the carpet is a lot harder now. Standing up and bending over can trigger bouts of dizziness, and just walking across the room can leave you short of breath. Errands become bigger productions, too. Just getting ready to go to the grocery store can sap your energy, and fighting crowds makes it worse.

Many people with COPD rely on family members and friends to take over responsibility for most household chores. Eventually, you may need a personal aide to help you with basic activities like bathing and grooming, or even a home health aide to help you with medications and exercises.

Losing it emotionally

The progressive nature of COPD and the continually shrinking limits on your activity put a huge burden on your emotional and mental reserves. Depression and anxiety disorders are much more common in COPD patients than in the general population: Whereas less than a third of the general population suffers from these disorders, nearly half of all COPD patients do.

Men and women both can develop depression and other mood or emotional problems, but women seem to be more vulnerable to them. Studies have found that women have a more pessimistic attitude toward being able to control their COPD symptoms and are more likely to report that their COPD has lowered their quality of life.

A number of factors contribute to the emotional effects of COPD. If you're a smoker or former smoker, you may feel guilty about "bringing this on yourself," or you may find that others are less sympathetic or understanding of your symptoms because they believe it's your own doing.

Having to give up work can inflict its own emotional torture. So many people wrap their sense of self and value around their occupations that the withdrawal from the working world can leave them feeling empty and even worthless.

Having to rely on family and friends to do the routine household tasks you can no longer do may spark resentment and make feelings of worthlessness more intense. Most people don't want to become a burden to their loved ones and will grapple with guilt and other negative feelings as they become more dependent on others.

Finally, fear is a formidable force when you have COPD. You may worry about what will happen when your disease progresses to the point where you can no longer take care of yourself. You may fear having a sudden attack and worry about how it will affect your overall health and quality of life. The list of potential fears and worries is virtually endless, and so is the potential for these fears and worries to cause extreme stress, another risk factor for worsening COPD symptoms.

Living with COPD is challenging both physically and mentally. Newly diagnosed patients often are overwhelmed and even confused about what their disease is and what can be done about it. The good news is that millions of Americans are living enjoyable, productive lives with COPD, and more attention is being paid to the treatments and effects of this once little-known and little-understood disease. With the ever-increasing wealth of resources available to you, including this book, you can manage your COPD so you can continue to enjoy life.

Chapter 2

How Your Lungs Work

*M*ost people don't think much about breathing until it becomes difficult — when they're exercising or when they come down with a cold, for example. When you have COPD, though, you suddenly find yourself thinking about your lungs in ways you never did before. You no longer take breathing for granted.

Knowing what's going on inside your body helps. The more you understand about how your lungs work, the better you'll be at figuring out how COPD is affecting you — and the easier it'll be for you and your doctor to come up with a treatment program that makes sense for you.

Breathing is an *involuntary function,* something your body does automatically. It's controlled by a complex set of organs and signals in your body that you aren't even aware of; you don't have to think about breathing to keep doing it. In fact, you couldn't stop yourself from breathing even if you wanted to. (Of course, unless you're a 10-year-old on a playground, holding your breath as long as you can to win a dare, you probably don't find it fun to try to stop yourself from breathing.) Assuming you could hold your breath long enough, you would lose consciousness and start breathing again, immediately and automatically.

In this chapter, we show you how your body takes in oxygen and gets rid of other gases, like carbon dioxide. We also describe the differences between healthy lungs and damaged lungs, and we discuss various factors that can affect how your lungs function.

Your Breathing System

Folded up inside your rib cage, your lungs look deceptively small. In fact, they're the second largest organ in your body (only the skin, which is also an organ, is larger). If you could lay them out flat, your lungs would cover a football field. They need all that surface area to efficiently allow oxygen into your body and carbon dioxide out of it.

That sounds simple enough, but your lungs are only one element in a sophisticated chain of organs that regulate your breathing (see Figure 2-1). The process of inhaling and exhaling also involves your:

- **Epiglottis:** A little flap of tissue that prevents food and liquid from going into your lungs when you swallow

- **Trachea (or windpipe):** The main airway that supplies both your lungs

- **Diaphragm:** The muscle that separates your chest cavity from your abdominal cavity

- **Intercostal muscles:** The muscles between your ribs

- **Bronchi:** The tubes that connect your windpipe to your lungs

- **Bronchioles:** The progressively tinier branches that extend deep into your lungs

- **Alveoli:** Little air sacs at the base of the bronchioles

- **Pulmonary capillaries:** Small blood vessels surrounding each air sac

- **Medulla, hypothalamus, and cortex:** Parts of the brain that regulate how fast you breathe

Your left lung is divided into two lobes, but your right lung has three. The left lung is smaller than the right lung, to accommodate the heart; it actually has a small impression where the heart rests against it. Each lobe in your lungs is surrounded by a membrane called a *pleura;* another pleura separates your lungs from the wall of your chest. The space between these membranes is normally filled with a small amount of fluid that prevents friction while you breathe.

Your diaphragm and intercostal muscles expand and contract as you breathe, helping your lungs take in and expel air. You can feel them at work by sitting up straight, placing your hands on your rib cage, and taking a deep breath. As you inhale, your ribs should push your hands outward, and your belly should expand, too. When you exhale, your ribs and abdomen should contract, helping force air out from the bottom of your lungs.

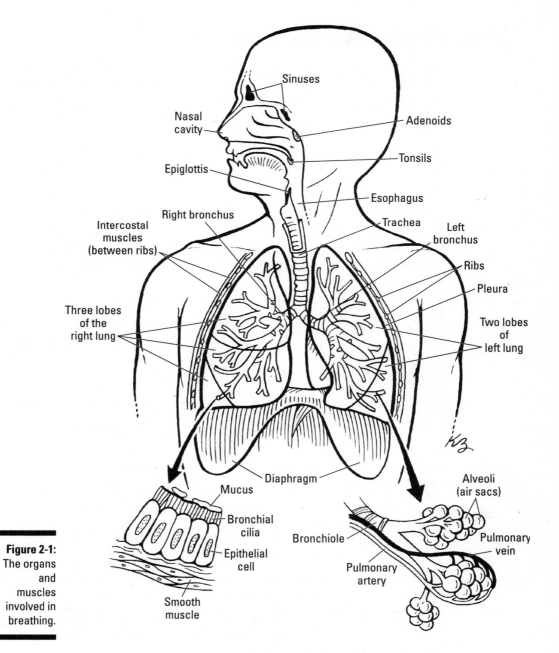

Figure 2-1:
The organs
and
muscles
involved in
breathing.

What happens when you breathe

Here's what happens when you take a normal breath: Air enters through your mouth or nose, the epiglottis opens to allow the air into your windpipe, and the air travels through the bronchi into the bronchioles, which look like the branches on an upside-down tree, getting smaller the farther into your lungs they go. (The bronchi and bronchioles together are often referred to as *bronchial tubes.*) At the end of each of these branches is a cluster of microscopic air sacs called *alveoli* that look like bunches of tiny grapes or soap bubbles. Each little sac — there are about 300 million of them in a healthy lung — is covered in small blood vessels.

When you inhale, the blood in the pulmonary capillaries is high in carbon dioxide and low in oxygen. The oxygen in the air you breathe in is absorbed from your air sacs into your blood, and the carbon dioxide in your blood is transferred into your air sacs. You then expel the carbon dioxide from your body when you exhale. And your blood carries its new load of oxygen to your heart, your brain, and the rest of your body. (This process, known as the *gas exchange,* because it's the exchange of oxygen for carbon dioxide, is illustrated in Figure 2-2.)

All this takes only a fraction of a second, and your body does it all on its own, an average of 15 to 25 times every minute while you're resting. That's because your medulla, hypothalamus, and cortex send and receive signals from your lungs and special cells throughout your respiratory system that continually monitor oxygen and carbon dioxide levels. And when you hold your breath, your brain sends a signal to your lungs ordering them to start breathing again.

Sensor cells

Your central nervous system has a variety of specialized cells that monitor the levels of oxygen and carbon dioxide in your blood. These cells send signals to your brain when the levels are out of balance. Some of these cells are located in your *aorta,* the largest artery in your body, which begins at your heart. Some are located in your *carotid arteries,* the arteries on either side of your neck that supply oxygen to your brain. Still others are located in your brain stem. The cells in the brain stem pay particular attention to the carbon dioxide level in the fluid that encompasses your brain and spinal cord. If too much carbon dioxide is in this fluid, your lungs receive a signal to increase the rate of breathing and to take in deep breaths. When the carbon dioxide level drops to an acceptable level, your breathing rate returns to normal.

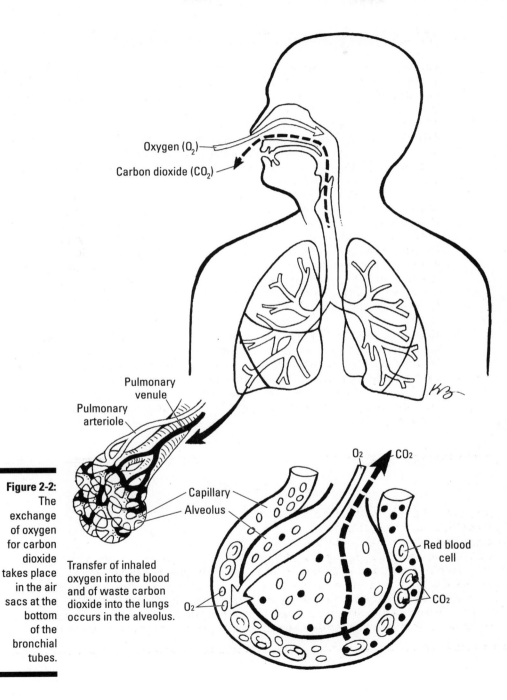

Oxygen (O$_2$)

Carbon dioxide (CO$_2$)

Pulmonary venule

Pulmonary arteriole

O$_2$ CO$_2$

Capillary

Alveolus

Red blood cell

CO$_2$

O$_2$

Figure 2-2: The exchange of oxygen for carbon dioxide takes place in the air sacs at the bottom of the bronchial tubes.

Transfer of inhaled oxygen into the blood and of waste carbon dioxide into the lungs occurs in the alveolus.

Your body's air filtration system

Your respiratory system does more than take in oxygen and expel carbon dioxide. It also performs sophisticated tasks to control the temperature and moisture content of the air you take in and to reduce or remove irritants in the air.

The process starts with the hairs inside your nose, which trap small particles of dust, pollen, and other irritants. When you get a good whiff of these particles, you get a tickling sensation that tells you to blow your nose or that causes you to sneeze. Sneezing is part of your body's defense system; it forces foreign matter out.

Your bronchial tubes also are lined with tiny hairs called *cilia*. These act like little brooms, sweeping back and forth to move *mucus* (the sticky substance you sometimes cough up, especially when you have a cold or allergies) out of the lungs and into the throat. Mucus is like a magnetic dust cloth, catching a lot (though not all) of the irritants that can invade the lungs, like dust and germs.

From your nose, air moves into your sinuses, which help regulate the humidity and temperature of the air you take in. As the air moves down into your windpipe, it passes two portions of your *lymph system* (part of the body's infection-fighting defenses): First are your *adenoids,* tissue at the top of your throat, followed by your *tonsils,* which are located in the walls of your throat. Both help to filter out foreign objects like germs, and both produce infection-fighting cells called *lymphocytes.* (The adenoids and tonsils are sometimes surgically removed if they become enlarged or frequently infected.)

Unless you're congested from a cold or allergies, you should try to breathe through your nose instead of through your mouth. Breathing through your nose lets your body take full advantage of its air filtering system. The exception is when you're exercising — then you should breathe through your mouth to increase the rate of gas exchange in your lungs.

Healthy Lungs versus Damaged Lungs

Even though they're inside your body, your lungs are primarily affected — arguably more than any other organ — by what's *outside* your body: the quality of the air you breathe, even down to the temperature and humidity. How well your lungs perform their jobs of gas exchange and air filtration depends on how healthy they are.

In the following sections, we show you the difference between healthy lungs and damaged lungs.

Healthy lungs

Healthy lungs (see Figure 2-3) are pink and porous like a sponge, springy to the touch. Like a balloon, they expand and then return to their original shape when air is expelled. This elasticity, coupled with the millions of tiny air sacs on your lungs' surface, allows you to pull in oxygen and get rid of carbon dioxide quickly and efficiently.

Healthy lungs also have a reserve capacity. Only rarely do people breathe deeply enough to fill their lungs completely, because only rarely do their bodies require such deep breaths. Normally, the action of the diaphragm pulls in enough air to sustain the body.

In fact, there are cells called *stretch receptors* in the lungs and chest wall whose job it is to keep people from overinflating their lungs. When you do breathe too deeply, these cells signal you to exhale; they may even tell you to breathe more slowly, so you don't damage your lungs by overstretching them.

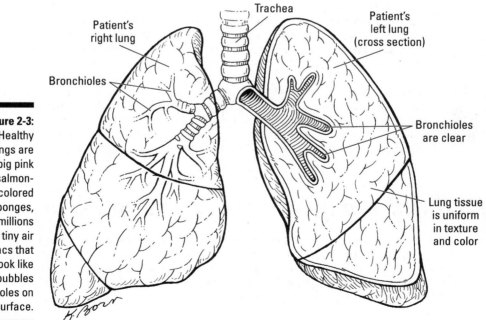

Figure 2-3:
Healthy lungs are like big pink or salmon-colored sponges, with millions of tiny air sacs that look like bubbles or holes on the surface.

Damaged lungs

When lungs get damaged, they may lose their ability to exchange oxygen for carbon dioxide, and that makes you feel short of breath. Damaged lungs (see Figure 2-4) aren't as elastic as healthy lungs, so they can't retain their original efficient structure. Airways may get narrower or collapse; picture a deflated balloon, like the long thin ones clown use to make balloon animals.

Sometimes the air sacs may stay inflated and trap air even when the airways leading to them collapse. That means you have to work harder to exhale the air you take in. (This situation is especially problematic during physical exertion, where you breathe fast and can't exhale adequately before it's time to inhale again.) And when the air sacs stay inflated, your lungs take up more room in your chest cavity, which can cause a full or tight sensation in your chest.

Sometimes the air sacs get destroyed or deformed, leaving only a relatively few, larger air sacs to send oxygen into the blood and take carbon dioxide out of it. This decreases the efficiency of the gas exchange because there's less surface area in which it can take place. As a result, you feel short of breath.

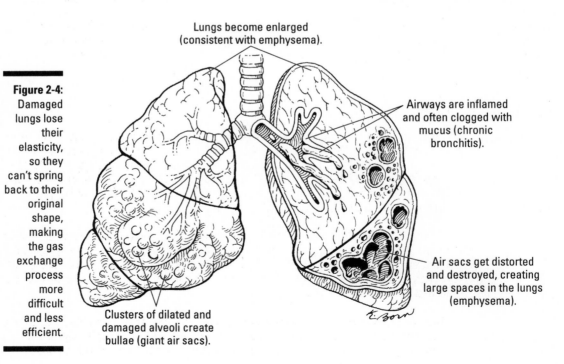

Lungs become enlarged
(consistent with emphysema).

Figure 2-4:
Damaged lungs lose their elasticity, so they can't spring back to their original shape, making the gas exchange process more difficult and less efficient.

Airways are inflamed and often clogged with mucus (chronic bronchitis).

Air sacs get distorted and destroyed, creating large spaces in the lungs (emphysema).

Clusters of dilated and damaged alveoli create bullae (giant air sacs).

Irritation can make the walls of the airways thicken and harden. It also may prompt your lungs to produce more mucus in an attempt to get rid of the irritant. When the airways are less flexible and clogged with extra mucus, it makes it that much harder to get air into and out of the lungs. The extra mucus also leads to more coughing, adding to the feeling that you can't catch your breath.

Because of the reserve capacity of your lungs, you probably won't be aware of damage to them right away. By the time most people see a doctor because they're feeling short of breath, the damage has progressed fairly far.

Factors That Influence Your Lung Function

A number of things affect how well your lungs work. One is genetics: A family history of lung problems may mean you're more susceptible to problems yourself. Depending on their severity, childhood diseases, allergies, and asthma can have an impact on how well your lungs carry on their job, too.

And then there are the factors that influence everyone to one degree or another. These include both the inevitable — getting older — and some things you *can* control, like exposure to certain irritants or smoking.

Age

For the first two decades of life, the body slowly but steadily creates new air sacs in the lungs. That activity stops around age 20, and from then on, the lungs lose tissue. The number of air sacs decreases as you age, and when the air sacs go, so do the blood vessels that surround them. That means there's less surface area to conduct the gas exchange, so the diffusion of oxygen through your blood is generally lower, too.

After you reach age 30 or thereabouts, your maximum lung function gradually drops. Normal breathing usually isn't noticeably affected, but your lungs may have trouble keeping up with extra demands. For example, returning to normal breathing after exercise takes longer, and it may not take much exertion at all to feel a little short of breath.

Your muscles and bones change as you age, too, and those changes can affect your breathing. Your diaphragm may become weaker, so it isn't as efficient at helping your lungs pull air in. The muscles between your ribs may lose strength, and your chest may not stretch as far or as easily as it did when you were younger. Bone problems like osteoporosis — especially when it involves the "hunchback" curving of the spine — or excess mineral deposits can make it more difficult to breathe. Your breathing pattern may change, too, in response to these issues; you may begin taking more shallow breaths more often, instead of taking slow, deep breaths.

Environmental factors

Your lungs interact with the environment with every breath. When you breathe in air, you also take in whatever is *in* the air — dust, soot, pollen and spores, noxious gases, and so on. Usually, your body's natural defenses (see "Your body's air filtration system," earlier in this chapter) can keep these foreign invaders at bay. But sometimes they overwhelm your defenses, and, when they do, they can cause real damage.

Dust

The term *dust* is a broad one, referring to tiny particles of some material that float in the air. Dust can come from organic or inorganic matter; hay and grain give off dust, as can metals like iron and tin, fuels like coal, and elements like silica or barium. Dust also comes from pet dander, hair, feathers, and even animal droppings.

Just as heavier particles of dust can settle on your furniture, they can settle in the air sacs in the bottom of your lungs. When they do, they're attacked by cells called *macrophages* that encompass the invader and carry it up to the cilia, where it can be swept up and out of the lungs.

Macrophages do an excellent job with most dust types, but they fail — and can cause permanent injury to the lungs — in some circumstances. For example, when they surround particles of silica dust, the macrophages die, emitting toxic material into the lungs. This can cause a buildup of scar tissue, which can interfere with lung function. When it reaches this stage, this condition is called *fibrosis*.

Most of the airborne dust you encounter on an everyday basis can be trapped easily by breathing through your nose; the hairs in your nose will catch these particles before they can get into your lungs. You can also minimize the impact of dust that does get into your lungs by taking quicker, shallower breaths.

Pollutants

Like dust, pollutants can be found indoors or out, and they can come from either biological or chemical sources. Biological sources of pollution include things like mold spores. Chemical sources include things like cleansers, car exhaust, and factory emissions.

Some pollutants contain tiny particles that, like dust, can be breathed in and can settle in your air sacs. Others can cause irritation — such as congestion, coughing, or sneezing — that makes it hard to breathe normally. These symptoms tell you that your body's defense system is working.

One especially potent pollutant is *ozone*. When it stays where it belongs — 6 miles or higher above the Earth's surface — ozone protects the planet from some of the harmful effects of the sun. But ground-level ozone, caused by a combination of chemical pollutants like car exhaust and strong sunlight, is a key ingredient in smog, and it can cause breathing problems even for people with healthy lungs. Because of the connection with strong sunlight, ozone warnings are more common in warmer months.

Because of its connection with smog, you may think urban areas are more likely to have ozone problems. But rural areas get their share of high-ozone days, too, largely because winds can carry ozone several hundred miles.

When you have COPD, be sure to limit your exposure to ground-level ozone by staying inside as much as possible on high-ozone days. Ozone can worsen the symptoms of bronchitis and emphysema, and prolonged exposure can cause additional scarring of the lung tissue.

Lifestyle factors

Your lifestyle also affects your lung function, because it helps determine what your lungs are exposed to every day. If you live in a big city and walk to work, chances are you're exposed to a great deal of car exhaust and other pollution. If you work on a farm, you may breathe in quite a bit of grain dust and other particles.

Two of the most important lifestyle factors, though, are smoking and exercise, or lack of it. The choices you make in these two areas can have a profound impact on how well your lungs work, regardless of whether you already have COPD or you're trying to avoid it.

Smoking

Cigarette smoking (and cigar and pipe smoking, if the smoke is inhaled) causes two problems for your lungs: It adds poisonous gases — such as carbon monoxide and nitrogen oxides — to the oxygen you take in when you breathe, and these gases get into your blood stream through the gas exchange process. By some estimates, cigarette smoke contains around 4,000 toxic chemicals, and more than 40 of them are linked to cancer. The smoke of an average cigarette contains, among many other things, formaldehyde (used to embalm dead bodies), arsenic (used in rat poison and murder mysteries), and ammonia (a common household cleanser).

Tobacco smoke also contains tiny particles that, by the nature of smoking, get pulled deep into your lungs, forming tar that damages your lung tissue. These chemicals and particles also can kill off the cilia in your lungs and promote the production of extra mucus, which in turn can clog your airways and give you the infamous "smoker's hack."

Secondhand smoke, or passive smoking, can actually be more dangerous because smoke inhaled this way doesn't pass through the filter on the cigarette. That means more of the harmful chemicals in tobacco smoke are free to enter your lungs, even if you've never taken a single puff on a cigarette yourself.

Lack of exercise

As noted in the "Age" section, earlier in this chapter, your lung function changes as you age. But regular exercise can help slow the effects of aging — and lack of exercise can make your lungs age faster.

There are several reasons for this:

- **When you don't exercise, you tend to gain weight.** The more weight you carry, the harder your respiratory system has to work to get oxygen into the blood. Any additional exertion can make this job even more difficult, causing you to get short of breath.

- **Lack of exercise usually means the muscles involved in breathing — particularly your diaphragm and the muscles between your ribs — will weaken, so you'll have a harder time drawing in deep breaths.** You may have a harder time expanding your chest wall, too, especially if you're carrying extra weight.

- **Failing to exercise may disguise the symptoms of serious lung trouble.** If you become short of breath after climbing a flight of stairs, you're likely to attribute the symptom to not being used to the exertion, and you probably won't seek medical attention for it until you find yourself short of breath even while resting.

How smoke attacks your lungs

Scientists have just recently discovered why cigarette smoke can be so harmful to the lungs. Cells in your body have little ports — tiny tunnels that lead from the center of the cell to the outer membrane — that they use to exchange chemical information and to change their own size and structure. Usually, cells have two of these ports, called *hemichannels.* But sometimes cells only have one port. When those kinds of one-port cells from the lungs and heart are exposed to cigarette smoke, the toxic chemicals have a direct route inside the cell, and helpful chemicals leak out. This exchange of toxins for needed and useful chemicals results in injury and even death of the cell.

Chapter 3

COPD Risk Factors

. . . .

In This Chapter

▶ Identifying your exposure risk

▶ Looking into your demographic risk

▶ Exploring the risks in your medical history

▶ Figuring out when to ask your doctor about your risk

. . . .

Risk factors for COPD come under three main headings: behavior, demographics, and medical history. Some of these things you can control; others you just have to accept as beyond your control. Either way, knowing your COPD risk factors helps you and your doctor evaluate and properly identify any lung problems you may have.

In this chapter, we look at all three kinds of risk factors. We show why these things increase your risk, and we give you tips on how to minimize the factors that apply to you.

You aren't necessarily doomed to COPD just because some of these risk factors apply to you. Individuals vary widely in their tolerance for and response to all kinds of risks. But even if you don't have any COPD symptoms, knowing how your behavior and background may affect your lung health can help you take preventive steps now. And because there is no cure for COPD, an ounce of prevention is absolutely priceless.

Risky Behaviors

When we talk about risky behaviors, we're not talking about things like forgetting to wear your seatbelt or spending your weekends skydiving. When it comes to the health of your lungs, risky behaviors are activities that expose your lungs to harmful gases, fumes, and dust — things that, over the course of many years, can cause permanent damage to your lungs.

Some of these behaviors are matters of personal choice, like smoking. Some are not; if you're a miner or construction worker or nurse, for example, some exposure to noxious elements is virtually inevitable. Even if you can't avoid all potentially risky behaviors, you can take steps to minimize your risk, when you know where the risk lies.

Smoking: The number-one risk

The correlation between smoking and COPD is exceptionally strong. As many as 90 percent of all COPD cases occur in people who currently smoke or who are former smokers. This doesn't mean you definitely will develop COPD if you are or once were a smoker. In fact, for reasons that still aren't clear to researchers, only about 20 percent of smokers are diagnosed with COPD. But because so many cases of COPD are linked to smoking, it is considered the single biggest risk factor for the disease.

If you started smoking at a young age, your risk for developing COPD is higher than it is if you started smoking when you were older. How long you've smoked and how much you've smoked also affect your risk level. If you've smoked three packs a day for 20 years, your risk is higher than if you've smoked five cigarettes a day for 10 years. If you smoked when you were younger but quit after a few years, your risk probably is lower than if you smoked for more than ten years before you quit.

Doctors and researchers use the term *total pack years* to help them figure out how high your risk of various lung diseases is. Total pack years equals the number of cigarettes or packs you smoke in a day, multiplied by the number of years you've been smoking. There are 20 cigarettes in a pack. If you smoke 2½ packs a day for 10 years, that's 25 pack years ($2.5 \times 10 = 25$). If you smoke 5 cigarettes a day, or a quarter-pack, for 10 years, that's only 2½ pack years ($0.25 \times 10 = 2.5$). The lower the number of pack years, the less damage you do to your lungs with smoking, although your doctor, of course, would prefer your pack-year number to be zero.

Your risk also is affected by whether you still smoke. If you've cut back, you're still at risk, but you probably aren't causing as much damage to your lungs as when you smoked full-bore. If you've quit, that's even better; even though you can't undo any lung damage that's been done, you stop adding to the damage when you cut out smoking completely. (See Chapter 10 for detailed information on kicking the habit.)

Even if you've never smoked a single cigarette, you may be at risk if you're around smokers a lot. Secondhand smoke can damage your lungs just as much as active smoking can. Indeed, some research indicates that second-hand smoke is more dangerous to your lungs because there is no filter to block out any of the harmful gases. If you spend a lot of time in smoky places like bars, your lungs could be suffering more than you know.

Pipe and cigar smokers have a higher risk for developing COPD than people who have never smoked, but the risk isn't as high as it is for current and former cigarette smokers. The difference may be in how you smoke: Pulling smoke deep into your lungs, as you do when you smoke cigarettes, is more damaging to your lungs than holding the smoke in your mouth or the upper part of your lungs, as most pipe and cigar smokers do. However, even if you don't inhale pipe or cigar smoke deeply, you do increase your risk of oral, throat, and other types of cancer.

Smoking marijuana alone hasn't been linked to COPD, but it has been shown to increase both the risk and symptoms of COPD in people who are current cigarette smokers. A Canadian study showed that smoking both cigarettes and marijuana created an eightfold increase in COPD risk.

On-the-job risks

Occupational hazards have been linked to many lung diseases, including COPD. Workers who are exposed to so-called "nuisance dust" (dust that the U.S. Occupational Safety and Health Administration defines as containing less than 1 percent silica and that, therefore, is not harmful to the lungs) are almost one and a half times more likely to suffer impaired lung function, and those who are exposed to high levels of dust are more than three and a half times more likely to develop symptoms of asthma or COPD. Even if you're a nonsmoker (meaning you have never smoked), if you're exposed to dust, fumes, or other pollutants at your job, you have a higher risk of developing COPD; the effects of inhaling dust are fully half the effects of smoking.

About 30 percent of COPD cases in people who have never smoked are attributed to occupational risks. And these hazards are of concern to smokers, too: For between 15 percent and 19 percent of smokers who have COPD, the disease can be traced to on-the-job exposure to harmful materials.

Working underground

The link between COPD and people who work underground — like coal or hard-rock miners, tunnel workers, and so on — is well-established. Workers in these occupations tend to breathe in dust from minerals like silica and quartz. This dust can settle deep in the lungs and cause inflammation and scarring. In some cases, your body's efforts to get rid of the mineral dust can release toxins into your lungs (see Chapter 2).

Working with metal

Working with metal creates tiny particles of metal dust that can be inhaled. Welding adds to the risk because you are exposed not only to metal dust but also to gases emitted by the welding machinery and gases that are created when metal heats up. Some research shows that prolonged exposure to welding fumes has much the same effect as smoking, even among people who have never smoked; add smoking to the mix, and the problem is just compounded.

Prolonged exposure to welding fumes has been linked to bronchitis. In fact, welding fumes are just as harmful to your lungs as smoking, according to some research, and the combination of welding fumes and smoking is even more damaging.

Even if you aren't a welder or a miner, you're exposed to potentially harmful metals every day in your diet, in the air you breathe, and in the products you use at work and at home. Cadmium, for example, is present in batteries, television components, solder, and even polyvinyl chloride (PVC). Industrial exposure to cadmium and other harmful metals has been reduced significantly over the past 50 years, but environmental and health experts agree that more needs to be done to minimize risks for workers and the general public. (See the nearby sidebar, "Cruel cadmium," for more on cadmium.)

Working around organic and biological dust

Occupations that expose you to dust from biological sources also can increase your risk for COPD. Plant fibers, pollen, bacteria, and *endotoxins* (toxic substances that are released when bacteria die) all can cause irritation, inflammation, and scarring in the airways and air sacs.

Farmers, grain handlers, sawmill workers, and cotton workers all are exposed to higher-than-average levels of organic or biological dust. So are bakers, hairdressers, and nurses. Women tend to be exposed to these dusts more often than men, while men tend to be more frequently exposed to mineral dust, gases, and fumes.

Dust from cotton can produce asthma-like symptoms and make you cough up phlegm or mucus. Grain and wood dust are associated with chronic bronchitis, declines in lung function, and even *occupational asthma* (asthma created through working conditions).

Other occupations

COPD has been linked with several specific occupations, generally because of the higher exposure to dust and fumes that irritate the lungs and lead to scarring of the airways. Jobs associated with higher prevalence of COPD include:

- Construction
- Factory work, especially leather, rubber, and plastics
- Textiles, such as cotton workers and weavers
- Food products (processing and manufacturing)
- Spray painting

Cruel cadmium

Cadmium is a particularly nasty metal when it comes to COPD and your general health. Inhaling cadmium dust and fumes irritates the airways, which can lead to scarring and deformation of the air sacs. Cadmium fume exposure has been associated with emphysema and is up to twice as harmful as coal dust. Ingesting cadmium through contaminated meat or farm products can cause stomach and kidney problems. And your body isn't very good at ridding itself of cadmium, so low-level exposure over several years can lead to stomach and kidney problems as well

as COPD. For nonsmokers, the most common ways of getting cadmium into the body are by eating plants that have grown in cadmium-contaminated soil and by breathing in dust from mining or manufacturing facilities. Cadmium also is present in cigarettes and marijuana, and most experts agree that, if you smoke, your average daily intake of cadmium is double that of a non-smoker. Part of the reason for this is that your lungs are much better at absorbing cadmium than your stomach is.

- ✓ Welding
- ✓ Concrete manufacturing
- ✓ Non-mining industrial work

Air quality

The quality of the air you breathe affects your risk for developing COPD, and it doesn't just apply to the air outdoors. The air in your home, your office, your car — anywhere, really — can be laden with particles, gases, and fumes that can irritate your lungs and make breathing more difficult. Prolonged exposure can, in turn, lead to scarring, narrowing of the airways, and deformation or destruction of the air sacs.

Mold and mildew are prime irritants and can pose problems indoors and out. Fumes from painting, household cleaners, and even cooking oils can hurt your lungs. Heating fuel — especially wood and kerosene — can give off smoke, fumes, and tiny particles that can irritate your lungs.

Make sure the room you're working in is properly ventilated when painting, cleaning, cooking, or heating your home. Fresh, circulating air helps dilute the concentration of harmful dust and fumes, so you don't take so much of them into your lungs.

Outdoors, vehicle exhaust, fumes from industrial sites, dust from grain elevators, and high levels of ozone are dangers. Again, prolonged exposure can permanently damage your lungs.

Gender, Age, and Economic Status

Researchers have linked demographic factors to the risk of developing COPD, although the reasons for these links aren't always clear. For years, it was assumed that men and women had roughly the same risk, for example, but now it appears that women are at higher risk. Because COPD is pretty uncommon in people younger than 40, age is a factor in this disease. And your economic status can add to or decrease your risk, depending on a number of related factors.

Why women are more susceptible to COPD

Recent research indicates that merely being female puts you at higher risk for COPD. This could be so for a number of behavioral, genetic, and environmental reasons. Women now are more likely than men to smoke, for instance, and smoking is a major factor in COPD. Women also seem to be more susceptible to the harmful effects of smoking, possibly because their lungs and airways are smaller than men's, so they get a bigger jolt per puff of the toxic elements in cigarette smoke.

Genetic factors may also make women more susceptible. Women's immune systems may respond differently than men's to the assault of cigarette smoke. This may be true of environmental factors, too; women's lungs may be more sensitive to dust, ozone, and other airborne irritants. This seems to be particularly true of biological dust (see "Working around organic and biological dust," earlier in this chapter). A recent study found that, in women, there is a significant link between exposure to biological dust and chronic bronchitis, emphysema, and COPD. No such link was found in men.

Certain women-dominated occupations have high exposure risk to biological dust: artists (who come in contact with textiles, animal-hair brushes, and other tools), cleaners (who are exposed to animal hair and dander, plant dust, and so on), food workers, textile workers, and healthcare professionals like nurses and home health aides.

The statistics for women with COPD are discouraging. Nonsmoking women are more likely than nonsmoking men to develop COPD. Women develop the disease at younger ages than men do, and they feel the severe effects of it earlier than men do. Women with COPD are more likely than men with the same severity of the disease to describe themselves as depressed and to rate their quality of life as poor. More women than men seek emergency medical care for their symptoms, and more women than men die from COPD each year.

Men do fare worse than women in some areas, especially when it comes to mild COPD. Men with mild COPD are more likely to lose weight and see a drop in their ability to exercise or otherwise be active, while women don't see these effects until the disease progresses to the moderate or severe level. For reasons that aren't yet fully understood, men who are on oxygen therapy live longer than women on oxygen therapy.

Overall, though, COPD strikes women harder. Recent studies showed that, even when COPD was at the same level of severity in both men and women, women had lower lung function, more difficulty breathing, and poorer nutritional status than their male counterparts.

Why COPD generally strikes after age 40

COPD is the result of years of exposure to smoke, industrial pollutants, and other irritants that cause repeated damage to the lungs, suppressing the body's ability to defend itself and promoting scar tissue that interferes with lung function. Add this continual irritation to the natural decline of aging lungs (see Chapter 2), and it makes sense that COPD is more common in people who are 40 or older. In fact, the older you get, the more likely it is — depending on other risk factors, of course — that you'll develop COPD. Occasionally, younger patients are diagnosed with the disease, but these cases are rare and usually involve some exceptional circumstances.

Asthma patients — especially those who smoke or who have high exposure to noxious fumes, dust, and other irritants on the job — tend to be diagnosed with COPD at earlier ages than non-asthmatic patients.

Why low-income patients are at risk

Worldwide, COPD is more common among low-income patients than among those with higher incomes. This could be because low-income patients are more likely to be smokers than higher-earning individuals. There also could be an environmental explanation: Poor people tend to be exposed to more environmental hazards than wealthier people. The use of wood or oil for heating, for example, tends to be more prevalent among low-income households; mold and mildew are more common in older, poorly maintained housing; and low-income neighborhoods tend to have higher concentrations of airborne pollutants and dust particles.

Low-income patients also may delay seeking medical care, either because they have little or no health insurance coverage and little, if any, means to pay for treatment themselves, or because they lack access to qualified medical care because of transportation issues, inability to take time off from work, or other obstacles. The delay in diagnosis and treatment means the disease progresses further and the symptoms are more debilitating and harder to treat.

Looking Back: Heredity and Medical History

Genetics, your family's medical history, and your own medical history all can influence your overall risk for developing COPD. Not all of these are fully understood, and some of the potential risks may be canceled out by protective factors — and some of those protective factors you and your doctor may never be aware of, especially if they're genetic. There's very little you can do about your hereditary risk. However, knowing the possible risks in your broad medical history should motivate you to do what you can to minimize the risk factors you can control.

The genetic link to COPD

Researchers are far from understanding the complex and sophisticated ways in which various genes influence our overall health, much less how they operate when it comes to specific health problems. Most researchers believe that many genetic factors are involved in protecting us (or not) from developing COPD. When it comes to smoking, for example, researchers believe there is some genetic reason why four out of five smokers will never be diagnosed with COPD — or, conversely, some genetic factor that strikes one in five smokers and leads to COPD. Some genes that are suspected to play a role in COPD are also associated with inflammation processes; efforts to isolate these genetic factors have met with mixed results.

There is one well-documented genetic risk: a deficiency of a protein called *alpha-1 antitrypsin* (AAT), which is produced by the liver and plays a crucial role in protecting your lungs. Without this protein, emphysema is virtually a certainty; symptoms usually show up when patients are in their 30s or very early 40s. AAT-deficient people who smoke almost always have symptoms of lung disease — COPD or other disease — at an earlier age than either non-smokers with AAT deficiency or smokers who don't have this condition.

AAT deficiency is rare; only about 100,000 people in the United States have it, and it accounts for less than 5 percent of all emphysema cases in this country. However, an estimated 116 million people worldwide — including 25 million Americans — carry the gene that causes AAT deficiency, and these people can pass on the condition to their children.

Blood tests can determine whether you're a carrier of AAT deficiency or whether you have this condition yourself. A less invasive DNA test, involving a simple cheek swab, also has been developed to diagnose AAT deficiency.

If you're not yet 40 and your ability to exercise has decreased significantly or you often find yourself feeling short of breath, ask your doctor if you should be tested for AAT deficiency. A family history of early emphysema also may warrant testing to rule out AAT deficiency.

What your family history says about your COPD risk

There is some debate about whether a family history of COPD automatically increases your risk for developing it. Some studies have shown a strong correlation; others have not. However, given the suspected genetic factors in increasing or decreasing your risk for COPD, it makes sense to take into account your family's medical history.

Overall, *familial clustering* (which is what scientists call family history) of lung disease is a good sign that you should take particularly good care of your lungs. If a first-degree relative (a parent or full sibling) has chronic bronchitis, emphysema, or COPD, chances are, you're at higher risk of developing it. As you get out farther on the branches of your family tree, your risk from familial clustering generally decreases: Your risk is higher if your mother has COPD than if your grandmother had it, for example.

 For many years, doctors believed that COPD struck mainly Caucasian men in their 60s. More recent research, though, indicates that (a) women have a higher basic risk than men, (b) COPD in non-Caucasians may be overlooked or misdiagnosed, and (c) the average age of diagnosis is 53. If you're concerned about your risk, especially if you're in your mid-40s, ask your doctor whether it makes sense to take a *spirometry test* (a test that measures your lungs' air capacity).

What your own medical history says about your COPD risk

Factors from your childhood, your lifestyle as an adult, even what happened to you in the womb can influence your COPD risk. If you experienced severe respiratory infections as a child, your lungs may have suffered permanent damage, which can make the onset of COPD more likely. If your parents smoked in the house when you were a child, your lungs may have suffered from the effects of secondhand smoke. And if your mother smoked when she was pregnant with you, that may have affected the development of your lungs, which, in turn, could raise your risk for COPD.

Childhood lung diseases

Severe respiratory infections can cause permanent scarring in the lungs. When this scarring occurs, it interferes with the normal growth and development of your lungs. Childhood asthma also may affect your lung function as an adult.

Airway hyper-responsiveness

In everyday terms, this means your lungs become super-sensitive to irritants that other people can tolerate without symptoms. When you have this condition, you may develop a persistent cough, often with increased mucus, in response to irritants like mold, pollen, ozone, dust, or other forms of air pollution. Both asthma and airway hyper-responsiveness are considered risk factors for COPD.

Childhood exposures

Chronic exposure to secondhand smoke, noxious fumes, car exhaust, mold and mildew as a child can lead to reduced lung function and lung disease, including COPD, as an adult. These childhood exposures also can lead to airway hyper-responsiveness.

Lung growth

If your lungs didn't develop properly or fully in the womb, your maximum lung function will be reduced, and that increases your risk for COPD. Low birth weight and childhood exposures also can affect lung growth and development, which in turn may increase your risk for COPD.

Other possible risk factors

Research is uncovering links between COPD and several factors that don't, on the surface, seem like they should be related to lung function or disease. For example, some studies show that people who have periodontal disease — bleeding gums, infections, and so on — have a 50 percent higher risk of developing COPD than people with healthy gums. Why this should be so hasn't been determined, but gum disease also has been shown to be a marker for heart problems, so oral health may be an indicator of what's going on in the rest of your body.

Another factor is skin wrinkles, especially in smokers. A recent study found that deep wrinkling in middle-aged smokers was a reliable indicator that COPD was present, even if it hadn't been diagnosed yet. The link between wrinkling and COPD remained even after the researchers adjusted for smoking habits, sun exposure, and other variables.

Finally, diet and nutrition can be risk factors for COPD. Studies have shown that a diet high in fat, processed grains, and sugar increases your risk for COPD by a factor of five, while a diet rich in fruits, vegetables, and whole grains cuts your risk of developing COPD in half.

Assessing Your Risk

All this information about risk factors can be overwhelming, especially if several factors apply to you to one degree or another. Before you get too worked up, read the following questions and answer yes or no. This will give you a quick idea of whether you just need to be aware of your risks, or whether it's time to make an appointment with your doctor.

✔ Are you a current or former smoker?

✔ Have you smoked (or did you smoke) for more than ten years?

✔ Do you cough nearly every day?

✔ Do you cough up mucus most of the time?

✔ Do you expect to get bronchitis at least once every winter?

✔ Do you get colds that last several weeks instead of seven to ten days?

✔ Are you 40 or older?

If you answered yes to three or more of these questions, make an appointment with your doctor to discuss your concerns about COPD and set up the appropriate tests.

Part II
Catching Your Breath: Treating COPD

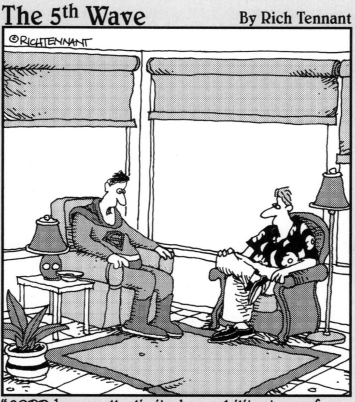

The 5th Wave   By Rich Tennant

"COPD has really limited my ability to perform the simplest activities. I can hardly scale a doghouse in a single bound, let alone tall buildings."

In this part . . .

There is no cure for COPD, but it can be managed and its progress can be slowed with proper care. In this part, we tell you about how COPD is diagnosed and how your doctor figures out whether you're "at risk" or whether you've got mild, moderate, or severe COPD. We also tell you about the emotional effects you and your loved ones may experience when COPD is diagnosed, and we give you strategies for dealing with those effects.

Managing COPD well involves all aspects of your physical and mental health, so we give you detailed information on building your healthcare team and setting treatment goals. And we present the latest information about various medications, therapies, surgeries, and alternative treatments — what you can expect them to do for you, the pros and cons of each treatment option, and questions you should ask your healthcare team.

Chapter 4

The Diagnosis and What It Means

COPD can be — and, alas, often is — mistaken for a number of other ailments, particularly asthma. The symptoms of COPD and asthma are similar, though with important differences; in fact, the courses of treatment use some of the same medications. But the proper treatment for COPD differs in important ways from the proper treatment of asthma.

That's why getting a correct diagnosis is so important. Your doctor should take a full medical history from you that covers any symptoms you have, your family history, and exposure to chemicals, dust, or other pollutants that are known to cause COPD (see Chapter 3). Then she should perform the appropriate tests to rule out other health issues and confirm the presence of COPD.

In this chapter, we tell you about the various tests used to diagnosis and assess the severity of COPD, including how they work, what they measure, and how you can prepare for taking these tests. We also look at other lung diseases and how your doctor will rule them out, and describe the various stages of COPD and the symptoms and limitations you can expect with each.

Finally, we break down exactly what your doctor can and cannot do to help you, and what you can do to help yourself. There is no cure for COPD, but it can be managed and its progress can be slowed with proper care.

Knowing Which Tests Your Doctor May Run

Many things can make you feel short of breath; COPD is just one of them. Your doctor may run — or order — several tests to rule out other causes and confirm the presence of COPD. Most of these tests are noninvasive and easy to perform. Some, like spirometry, may be performed right in your doctor's office. Others may have to be done at a separate lab, hospital, or imaging facility.

Spirometry testing

Spirometry is a simple test that provides your doctor with a wealth of information about your lung function and, indeed, many other aspects of your health. Even though it's a lung test, abnormal results can indicate problems with your heart or circulatory system.

How it works

A spirometer consists of a mouthpiece, a small chamber, and a hose hooked up to a computer that reads the measurements. You inhale deeply and put your lips tightly around the mouthpiece, forming a seal so all the air you exhale goes into the spirometer chamber. Then you take as deep a breath as you can and exhale as hard as you can for as long as you can. The spirometer measures how much air you force out of your lungs. (Figure 4-1 shows a patient doing a spirometry test.)

Ideally, you should be able to exhale for 6 seconds or more. Usually, you'll do this three times to ensure that the results can be reproduced (and, thus, considered accurate); your highest numbers will be used to evaluate your condition.

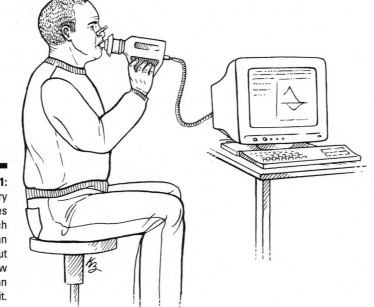

Figure 4-1:
Spirometry
measures
how much
air you can
blow out
and how
fast you can
exhale it.

To get the best reading out of your spirometry test, you shouldn't smoke for at least four to six hours before taking the test. Also, don't eat a heavy meal before the test. If you take any inhaler or bronchodilator medications, ask your doctor whether you should take them as usual before the test.

What it measures

Spirometry measures how much air you can force out of your lungs and how fast you can force it out. The first measurement is called *forced vital capacity* (FVC) and the second is called *forced expiratory volume* (FEV).

Your doctor will look at how much air you can force out in 1 second, called FEV1. FEV1 is the most common numerical value used to gauge the presence and severity of COPD.

What normal readings are

Your FEV and FVC vary according to your age, height, race, and gender. Young, tall, white males tend to have higher readings than older, shorter, white females, and African Americans and Asians of both sexes tend to have lower readings than their white counterparts. Lots of other variables may be in play, too. So spirometry readings are interpreted according to what's expected in an average person of your demographic group.

Your spirometry results are expressed as a "percentage of predicted," where *predicted* means what's expected as an average reading. Generally, normal readings are an FEV1 that's 80 percent or more of the predicted rate.

Even if you don't have trouble breathing (or don't think you do), you may consider having a spirometry test if you're a current or former smoker and you're 44 or older. You also should ask your doctor about it if you have a family history of COPD or long-term exposure to pollution or irritants.

How it detects COPD

Although spirometry can detect several different health issues, COPD gives characteristic readings that are different from other diseases like asthma. When you have COPD, your FVC — the total amount of air you exhale — is lower, and so is the amount of air you can exhale in 1 second (the FEV1 reading). But the real identifier is the ratio between the FEV1 and FVC, or how much air you exhale in the first second as a percentage of the total amount of air you exhale.

In healthy lungs, between 70 percent and 75 percent of all the air exhaled is exhaled in the first second. Various kinds of lung disease and airway obstructions can cause the FEV1 to be lower, but the ratio between the FEV1 and FVC remains fairly stable; that is, even if you're only able to take in a small amount of air with these other diseases, you still expel most of it in the first second of exhalation.

But when you have COPD, the FEV1-to-FVC ratio falls below 70 percent. In other words, you take the same amount of air in, but you can't get it out — the very essence of COPD.

Bronchodilator reversibility

If your initial spirometry readings are below normal, your doctor probably will have you inhale a bronchodilator and take the spirometry test again to see whether your lung function improves. If it does, that indicates the obstruction of your airways can be at least partially reversed with bronchodilators — hence, the name of the test.

An improvement of 12 percent or higher in the spirometry readings and an increase of 200 cubic centimeters (CCs) in your FEV1 after taking a bronchodilator indicates that your lung problem meets the guidelines for reversibility — that is, your condition is at least partially reversible with medication. Significant reversibility is seen in only a minority of COPD patients, but it's much more common in asthma patients. Doctors also sometimes use this method to evaluate the effectiveness of steroid treatment, usually a few weeks after you start taking steroids.

Diffusion capacity

When you have COPD your lungs aren't able to transfer oxygen into your blood as easily. Diffusion capacity testing tells your doctor how effectively the gas exchange between your air sacs and your bloodstream is working (see Chapter 2 for information on gas exchange).

For this test, you'll have clips put on your nose, and you'll be given a mouthpiece that fits tightly around your lips. You inhale a small (and safe) amount of carbon monoxide, hold your breath for a count of ten, and then exhale as hard as you can into a machine that measures how much of the carbon monoxide remains in the air you exhaled.

Low diffusion capacity can indicate the presence of severe emphysema, as well as other lung diseases.

Oximetry

Another way to figure out how much oxygen your lungs are transferring to your bloodstream is through a test called *oximetry*. This is usually done while you're exercising or while you're sleeping; it helps your doctor decide whether you would benefit from oxygen therapy.

Normal oxygen saturation is 95 percent or higher. With oximetry, the level of oxygen in your blood is determined by measuring how much light is transmitted through an area of your skin; to get an accurate reading, the device also has to be able to measure your pulse. It's noninvasive and usually does not cause much, if any, discomfort.

Although it's less invasive and less uncomfortable, oximetry is not as accurate as arterial blood gas testing (see "Arterial blood gas tests," later in this chapter). For the sake of detailed readings, your doctor may prefer to order the arterial blood gas test.

Lung volume tests

Lung volume is how much air your lungs can hold. If your doctor suspects COPD, she'll be interested in two specific measurements:

- **Total lung capacity (TLC):** How much air your lungs can hold. A high TLC indicates that the lungs are overinflated, which is common with emphysema.

- **Residual volume:** How much air remains in your lungs after you exhale. A high residual volume means you aren't getting air out of your lungs; the air is trapped, often in the bottom of the lungs.

Lung volume can be measured with a gas dilution test, similar to the diffusion capacity test (discussed earlier in this chapter) but using helium or nitrogen instead of carbon monoxide. A more accurate test is called *body plethysmography*. In this test, you sit in an airtight chamber (which is usually made of transparent glass or plastic so you don't get claustrophobic) and breathe in and out into a tube. The device measures pressure changes to determine the volume of air in your lungs.

Like spirometry, normal lung volume readings depend on your age, height, gender, and race. Your doctor looks at both the actual numbers and the percentage of predicted volume for your demographic group to see how your lungs compare. Higher-than-expected readings show that there's some obstruction that prevents you from getting air out of your lungs.

Chest X-rays

Chest X-rays aren't terribly good as a diagnostic tool for COPD unless the disease is fairly advanced. However, your doctor may order one to help him rule out other diseases. When COPD is detectable by X-ray, the doctor typically will find signs like a flattened diaphragm, overinflated lungs, and *bullae* (large, deformed air sacs).

Neither a chest X-ray nor a physical exam can detect COPD in its early stages, when it's easiest to manage. If you or your doctor suspect COPD, insist on a spirometry test; it's the only test that is known to detect COPD early on.

Arterial blood gas tests

Arterial blood gas (ABG) tests are among the most invasive and uncomfortable tests for COPD, because they require drawing blood from an artery instead of from a vein, as is usually done. The blood has to be taken from an artery to get an accurate assessment of the gas exchange in your body.

For this test, the blood likely will be drawn from an artery in your wrist, or possibly the inside of your arm above your elbow. Arterial blood also can be drawn from the femoral artery in your groin.

Arteries are deeper in your body than veins, and they're surrounded by more nerves than veins are. That's why drawing arterial blood hurts more than taking blood from a vein does.

The gases in the arterial blood are measured to find out how much oxygen is in your blood, as well as how much of your *hemoglobin* (the oxygen-carrying part of red blood cells) is saturated with oxygen. The test also measures levels of carbon dioxide and blood pH.

Your doctor can use the results of this test to decide whether you need oxygen therapy. The carbon dioxide measurement also gives a clue about your overall lung function and your ability to *ventilate,* which is a fancy way of describing your body's ability to maintain normal carbon dioxide levels in your blood. If the readings are abnormal, your doctor may prescribe oxygen therapy; how much and how often will depend on your condition.

ABG tests also may be used to see if your oxygen therapy should be adjusted and how well the treatment for your COPD is working. When you're in the hospital, an ABG test may be done to see if you're getting enough oxygen.

Your doctor must know about any medications you're taking, including over-the-counter medicines like aspirin or cold remedies, and any vitamins, nutritional supplements, and herbal preparations. If you're allergic to any anesthetics, or if you're taking blood thinners like aspirin or Coumadin, be sure to let your doctor know *before* the test.

If you are on oxygen therapy and can breathe without it, your oxygen may be removed about 20 to 30 minutes before the blood for the ABG test is drawn. If you can't breathe without supplemental oxygen, you'll continue to receive oxygen without interruption.

By itself, an ABG test only shows whether your blood gas levels are normal. It can't determine the reason for abnormal readings, and low levels can be caused by a number of health issues. So it is most useful in combination with other tests that can positively identify COPD as the culprit.

Conditions like anemia can affect how much oxygen your blood carries, so ABG results need to be put in context with all other health data for each patient. Fevers or *hypothermia* (unusually low body temperature) also can throw off the readings. If you smoke or breathe in highly polluted air before the test, the readings will be less accurate. Breathing in things like carbon monoxide, secondhand smoke, and even the fumes from paint or varnish can affect the results; in fact, your doctor may reschedule the test under these conditions because the results would be more or less useless.

Ruling Out Other Lung Diseases

According to the National Institutes of Health, COPD is severely under-diagnosed; as many as 12 million Americans may have it and don't know it yet. In addition, lots of people with COPD have been misdiagnosed with asthma or other lung ailments, which means that, even though they may be seeing their doctor regularly, they aren't getting the appropriate treatment.

To make sure your diagnosis is correct, you and your doctor should work together to rule out other lung diseases. Your share of the work involves communicating your symptoms and medical history to your doctor. It helps, too, if you can identify symptoms associated with COPD and compare them with the symptoms of other lung problems.

Asthma

Most commonly, COPD is mistaken for asthma, mainly because coughing and wheezing are typical symptoms in both. However, there are clear differences between these two diseases:

✔ **Onset:** Asthma usually makes its first appearance in childhood or the teenage years; rarely does an adult with no previous history suddenly develop asthma. COPD, on the other hand, rarely develops before age 40 and is most often diagnosed in people who are in their 50s or 60s. (The exception to this is the young asthmatic smoker who has a family history of asthma; the presence of COPD can easily be overlooked in a patient like this.)

- ✔ **Exacerbations:** In asthma, sudden attacks usually are triggered by a specific circumstance: exercise, cold air, or allergens like pollen; when the trigger is removed, symptoms get better. In COPD, the most common cause for an *acute exacerbation* (sudden occurrence of very bad symptoms) is a respiratory infection like a cold or the flu. Although some things like secondhand smoke or high humidity can make COPD symptoms worse, removing the trigger usually doesn't, in itself, make the symptoms go away.

- ✔ **Symptoms in between exacerbations:** When asthmatics have the proper treatment, they often are symptom-free until something triggers an attack. In COPD, especially in the moderate to severe stages, symptoms never disappear entirely; they simply get worse during exacerbations.

- ✔ **Treatment:** Asthma can be treated with inhaled corticosteroids as a maintenance medication, and bronchodilators are prescribed to control symptoms if necessary or for acute attacks. For COPD patients, the proper treatment is the reverse: Bronchodilators are the maintenance medication to help keep airways open, and steroids, either in inhaled or pill form, are prescribed only when the bronchodilators aren't enough to manage the disease.

- ✔ **Reversibility:** In many cases, asthma is considered reversible because symptoms disappear on their own or with proper treatment. COPD is generally not reversible. Although symptoms can be treated (and some people may consider that to be "reversibility"), the damage done to lungs with COPD cannot be undone.

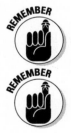

If you have a stuffy or runny nose along with your breathing problems, you're more likely to be suffering from *atopic asthma* (allergy-induced asthma) than from COPD. COPD patients rarely have allergies and, unless they also have a cold, they rarely have nasal symptoms along with their coughing and wheezing.

It's possible to have both asthma and COPD. When this happens, each disease makes the symptoms of the other worse and harder to control. Asthmatics who smoke are the most likely to suffer from both asthma and COPD.

Lung cancer

Lung cancer and COPD share a number of symptoms, and because smoking is the number-one risk factor for both, your doctor likely will order a variety of tests to positively identify what's ailing you.

Early-stage lung cancer, like early-stage COPD, presents either vague symptoms or none at all. You may find yourself becoming tired more easily and less inclined to choose a flight of stairs over an elevator, but, if you're like most people, these symptoms will not be severe enough to send you to your doctor.

By the time lung cancer and COPD cause symptoms bad enough to make you call your doctor, the disease is usually fairly advanced. Symptoms of lung cancer include

- Chronic cough
- Wheezing
- Coughing up blood
- Unexplained fever
- Weight loss
- Loss of appetite
- Hoarseness
- Shortness of breath
- Chronic bouts of bronchitis or pneumonia
- Chest pain

Except for the unexplained fever, chest pain, and coughing up blood, lung cancer and COPD symptoms are remarkably similar. If your doctor suspects lung cancer, he may order different tests. For example, if you're coughing up mucus, the doctor may have it tested for cancer cells. He may order a chest X-ray or CT scan, or a *bronchoscopy,* in which a small tube with a tiny camera attached is inserted through the nose or mouth and down the throat, allowing the doctor to see inside your airways and lungs. A tissue sample also may be taken during this procedure and *biopsied* (tested) for cancer.

If you're diagnosed with lung cancer, your doctor will order other tests to determine how advanced the cancer is and whether it has spread to other areas of the body. Treatment options depend on what the additional tests reveal.

Tuberculosis

Symptoms of tuberculosis, usually called TB, can mimic some COPD symptoms, but there are critical differences between these two diseases. Pulmonary TB — which accounts for three out every four TB cases — is an infection caused by bacteria; COPD is caused by the cumulative damage to the lungs caused by years of smoking, exposure to airborne irritants, or a genetic condition. Recently, there has been an increase in drug-resistant strains of TB; when COPD resists treatment, it's because the damage to the lungs is too far gone.

TB also often produces non-respiratory symptoms that are rarely present with COPD. Fever, chills, and night sweats are common TB symptoms — all indications of infection. COPD patients may sometimes have these symptoms, but only when they have an infection, not because of the COPD itself.

Pulmonary TB is contagious; COPD is *not*. With COPD, you don't have to take any special precautions to protect your family and others from your condition.

Pleurisy

Between your lungs and your chest wall are two thin membranes called the *pleura*. Usually, these membranes and the light coating of viscous fluid between them serve to lubricate the movements of your lungs against your chest wall. But they can get inflamed and infected. When that happens, every breath hurts because you no longer have that lubricating effect. Sneezing and coughing hurt even more. Such inflammation or infection is called *pleurisy* (or, more rarely, *pleuritis*).

Pleurisy is usually caused by a virus, but sometimes it's caused by another infection like pneumonia or TB. It also can be a secondary effect of other diseases like cancer, heart failure, rheumatoid arthritis, and kidney and liver disease. It may even occur as a reaction to certain medications. Pleurisy is usually treated by determining, and then treating, the underlying cause. Anti-inflammatory medications like ibuprofen help; sometimes steroids help reduce swelling in the pleura, too.

Assessing the Severity of Your COPD

You and your doctor can't design a treatment program for your COPD until you figure out how severe it is. If you're not bothered by symptoms on a regular basis, your doctor may prescribe a fast-acting bronchodilator for those times when you do have symptoms and otherwise focus on your overall health and lifestyle, outlining a diet and exercise program and urging you to quit smoking if you haven't already.

On the other hand, if your symptoms are so bad that you're unable to work, or even perform everyday tasks like cooking, bathing, and grooming, your treatment program will be much different.

The "at-risk" classification

If your spirometry tests are normal but you're a smoker or you work in a job where you inhale lots of dust or fumes, you're considered "at risk" for developing COPD. Your family history and your own medical background also can put you in the at-risk category (see Chapter 3 for a full discussion of things that can lead to COPD).

If you're at risk but don't actually have COPD yet, your doctor likely will recommend lifestyle changes that will reduce your chances of developing the disease. If you're a smoker, the first thing your doctor will tell you is to quit; she can help you figure out the method that will be most effective for you and prescribe medications to help with withdrawal symptoms. (See Chapter 10 for detailed information on smoking cessation methods.)

If you've already quit smoking or have never smoked, but you still have other risk factors for COPD, your doctor probably will recommend diet changes and an exercise program to help keep your lungs healthy.

Even if your first spirometry test is normal, you should be retested every three to five years. COPD and other lung diseases are progressive, so even if the damage isn't detectable now, it may show up later.

Mild COPD

Many people with mild COPD (sometimes called Stage I by doctors) don't get diagnosed because their symptoms are so subtle that they don't mention them to their doctors. You may feel a little out of breath if you do some hard physical labor, like raking the yard or lifting and carrying things, or when you walk fast. You may even notice that you can't do as much as you used to before you feel short of breath. And you may not think much of it, figuring that's only to be expected as you get older or put on a few extra pounds.

You also may cough more frequently than you used to. Sometimes you may cough up mucus, but probably not too often. Maybe you don't know why you cough, or maybe you figure it's just smoker's cough, especially if you do it most in the morning shortly after you wake up.

When COPD is mild, it usually doesn't interfere with your ability to work or carry out daily tasks like getting dressed, cooking, and cleaning. Treatment may be limited to diet and exercise if you don't suffer from acute exacerbations. In fact, diet and exercise may be the most effective ways to keep your COPD in the "mild" category; see Chapters 11 and 12 for information on how diet and exercise can affect your lungs.

From a medical standpoint, COPD is considered mild when your FEV1 (see the "Spirometry testing" section, earlier in this chapter) is higher than 50 percent of the predicted value for your age, height, gender, and race.

Your prognosis is best when COPD is detected in its mild stage. Long-term survival rates of people with mild COPD are only slightly lower than the survival rates of people who don't have COPD.

Moderate COPD

As COPD gets more severe, you feel its effects more. Coughing may be quite frequent, and you may cough up mucus more often. You get out of breath more often when you work hard or walk fast. You may even have a harder time doing chores like vacuuming or mowing the lawn. Even working at your job may be more tiring and difficult. And if you get a cold or chest infection, it may take you much longer to recover — as long as several weeks.

This is moderate (or Stage II) COPD, and it's when most people get concerned enough about their symptoms that they talk to their doctors. Your doctor may prescribe medications like bronchodilators to help keep your airways open. Diet and exercise also will be an important part of your treatment program (see Chapters 11 and 12).

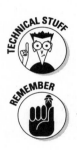

COPD is considered to be moderate when your FEV1 (see the "Spirometry testing" section, earlier in this chapter) is between 35 percent and 49 percent of the predicted value for your age, height, gender, and race.

No matter how severe your COPD is, quitting smoking is key to preventing further damage to your lungs. See Chapter 10 to find out how smoking harms your lungs and ways to approach the task of quitting.

Severe COPD

Stage III is the severest form of COPD. When it reaches this point, it interferes with your quality of life. Most people with severe COPD are unable to work; in fact, COPD is the second-leading cause of disability in the United States. You may cough many times every day, and you probably cough up a lot of mucus. You feel short of breath even when you're sitting or lying quietly; you may have so much trouble breathing at night that you try to sleep in a sitting or semi-reclined position. You're more susceptible than you used to be to colds and other infections, and you take much longer to get over them. You get tired extremely easily, and it's hard for you to even walk across the room, much less up a flight of stairs. You may feel weak, especially in your arms and legs, and you probably don't have much of an appetite, even if you're not fighting off a cold or infection.

COPD is considered severe when your FEV1 (see the "Spirometry testing" section, earlier in this chapter) is lower than 35 percent of the predicted rate for your age, height, gender, and race.

Treatment for severe COPD includes bronchodilators to help keep the airways open; corticosteroids also may be prescribed. (See Chapter 8 for a full description of the medications used to treat COPD.) Your doctor may order supplemental oxygen as part of your treatment to make breathing easier and make sure your body gets enough oxygen. Exercise and nutrition are as important in severe COPD as they are in other stages (see Chapters 11 and 12 for more on both).

The prognosis for severe COPD is poor. When FEV1 is less than 30 percent of the predicted value, nearly a third of COPD patients die within a year, and very few survive more than ten years. Because the lung damage cannot be reversed, treatment usually is focused on making you comfortable and improving your quality of life as much as possible.

Surgical procedures like *lung volume reduction surgery* and lung transplant may be considered for people with severe COPD (see Chapter 9 for details). Like other treatment options, these alternatives probably won't extend your life, but they can improve breathing and your quality of life.

Recognizing That There's No Cure, Only Care

When you develop COPD, you've got it for life; there is no cure. But, contrary to popular belief, COPD can be treated and managed. In fact, the only way to slow down the progression of COPD is to get proper treatment, which includes medication and making the right lifestyle choices — like quitting smoking, eating healthfully, and exercising regularly (see Part III of this book for more on all three of these).

Why lung damage can't be reversed

In general, the human body is pretty good at generating new tissue as it ages. But the lungs are one area where new cell growth stops pretty early in life, by the time you reach your 20s. You don't generate any new air sacs after that, and, as you get older, you actually lose air sacs — even if you haven't done anything, like take up smoking, to promote that loss. (See Chapter 2 for a full description of what happens to your lungs as you grow older.)

That's why lung damage can't be reversed. COPD is the cumulative result of long-term exposure to irritants that cause inflammation and scarring in your lungs. That's also why treatment of COPD focuses on preventing any further damage, and why we keep harping on the importance of quitting smoking. (We're not the only ones who will keep bringing this up; more than likely, your doctor will talk about it at every visit, and your family and friends may turn into nagging bores on the subject.)

Things you can do to feel better

The fact that COPD can't be cured doesn't mean you have to feel rotten all the time. You can do a number of things to feel better; in fact, the effectiveness of any treatment your doctor recommends will depend on how well you follow his instructions.

You'll find more information throughout this book on specific things you can do to feel better. Here's a quick checklist:

- ✔ Quit smoking. (We told you we were going to keep bringing this up.)
- ✔ Start exercising regularly.
- ✔ Add more fresh fruits and vegetables to your diet.
- ✔ Take your medications as prescribed.
- ✔ See your doctor every six months.

Things your doctor can do to help you feel better

Your doctor's arsenal of treatment options will depend in large part on how severe your COPD is and whether you have any other health issues that may affect treatment choices. The Global Initiative for Chronic Obstructive Lung Disease (GOLD) has issued treatment guidelines for COPD, ranging from identifying and evaluating COPD to treating severe or worsening symptoms:

- ✔ **Key indicators for COPD:** GOLD recommends that doctors consider COPD if patients 40 or older have any of these symptoms:

  - Shortness of breath that has gotten worse over time, that is present every day or nearly every day, or that gets worse with exercise

  - A chronic cough, even if it doesn't produce mucus and isn't present every day

  - Any chronic pattern of coughing up mucus

  - A history of exposure to risk factors (see Chapter 3)

- ✔ **FEV1 values for COPD stages:** FEV1 below 80 percent is considered mild; FEV1 between 50 percent and 80 percent is moderate; FEV1 between 30 percent and 50 percent is severe. FEV1 that's below 30 percent (or below 50 percent in conjunction with chronic respiratory failure) is considered very severe. (In all categories, the FEV1/FVC ratio is below 70 percent.)

The GOLD criteria, which are relatively new, list four levels of severity, but most American doctors are still accustomed to using the mild, moderate, and severe classifications we mention under "Assessing the Severity of Your COPD," earlier in this chapter. Because symptoms and treatment options are similar for both severe and very severe classifications, many doctors may not distinguish between the two except in your patient chart.

✔ **Therapy according to severity:** In mild COPD, the GOLD guidelines focus on reducing risk factors and preventing other illnesses like flu. When COPD is in the moderate stage, the guidelines call for adding long-acting bronchodilators as needed and pulmonary rehabilitation to maintain and maximize lung function. Inhaled steroids, oxygen therapy and possibly surgery are recommended for severe or very severe COPD.

✔ **Treating exacerbations:** When suddenly severe symptoms send a patient to the emergency room or require hospitalization, GOLD recommends ABG tests and chest X-rays, oxygen therapy, and the use of bronchodilators, steroids, and antibiotics as appropriate. The guidelines also call for carefully monitoring the patient's nutrition and hydration.

Assessing and monitoring

Your doctor will conduct a physical exam and ask about your medical history to assess your risk for COPD. She will order tests to rule out other possible causes like asthma (discussed earlier in this chapter) and try to assess how your symptoms affect you on a daily basis. She may ask you whether your symptoms ever get bad enough that you go to the emergency room, or whether you miss work, skip social functions, or feel anxious or depressed about your health and quality of life. She may also ask whether you've ever been *intubated,* or put on mechanical ventilation — what is commonly called "life support."

Reducing risk

This is where quitting smoking comes in. Your doctor also may advise you to avoid other risky things like exposure to fumes and chemicals. If your job exposes you to dust or fumes, your doctor may recommend changing your job duties or, if your symptoms are debilitating, going on disability. High humidity, high levels of ozone, and very hot or very cold temperatures also may make the list of things you should avoid.

Managing your symptoms

Diet, exercise, and medications all work together to keep your COPD symptoms under control and improve your quality of life. Be sure to take your medications exactly as directed and ask questions if you find any of the instructions confusing.

Your doctor may repeat various tests regularly to monitor the progress of your COPD and see if any of your medications should be changed. This is why it's important to see your doctor regularly; most experts recommend going every six months, even if you're feeling okay.

Preparing for sudden attacks

Sudden attacks, usually referred to as *acute exacerbations,* require special medications (see Chapter 8), often even hospitalization. Tell your doctor what happens when your symptoms suddenly get worse and how often you get such attacks. This information is a critical part of monitoring the progress of your COPD.

Keeping the treatment appropriate

If your COPD gets worse, your doctor may want to change your medication or adjust the dosage of the medicines you're already taking. He also may want to do additional testing to compare current results with previous readings. If you have an infection that makes your COPD worse, your doctor may want to put you in the hospital to make sure your condition is monitored and treated appropriately.

Chapter 5

The Emotional Impact of COPD

*I*f you're feeling down about your COPD and life in general, it may help to know you're not alone. A Canadian study found that about half of COPD sufferers also fit the criteria for psychiatric disorders, mainly depression and anxiety disorders. That compares with less than a third of the general population.

Women with COPD are more vulnerable to anxiety, depression, and other mood or psychiatric disorders than men, even when the severity and symptoms of their conditions are similar. The study found that, compared with male COPD patients, female COPD patients were more likely to have at least one psychiatric disorder, more likely to have been diagnosed with major depression at some point in their lives, and more likely to suffer from phobias, panic disorders, and anxiety disorders.

Women also tend to be less confident that their symptoms can be controlled and report that their symptoms have a greater impact on their quality of life than men.

That doesn't mean men with COPD are immune from its emotional effects, of course. Nearly four in ten male COPD patients met the criteria for a psychiatric disorder, and one in five had an anxiety disorder.

The study didn't establish a cause-and-effect relationship between COPD and depression, but it makes sense that chronic ill health can color your mental outlook. You may feel as though you're losing your independence and your ability to do the things you used to enjoy. You may worry about being a burden to your family and friends. If you're a current or former smoker, you may feel guilty about the damage that your habit did to your body, or you may feel (and, unfortunately, others may agree) that you don't deserve empathy for your health status now.

It's important to understand and deal with how you feel about your COPD and all the stuff that goes along with it, because your mental health can have a profound impact on your physical health. In this chapter, we take you through the emotional quagmire many COPD patients must navigate. We can't help you avoid it, but we can, and do, offer tips on getting through it.

Now What Do I Do?

It's not uncommon to feel a little confused and even panicky when your doctor tells you that you have COPD. The fact that there is no cure only adds to your distress; you may feel hopeless, as though the only thing you can do is go home and wait to die.

Of course, that's *not* all you can do. You can take control of your life with COPD by eating right, exercising as your doctor directs, taking your medications properly, and adjusting your routine to make everyday living easier. But first you have to get yourself past the initial shock and despair so you can find the answers to that pesky question, "Now what?"

Identifying your limitations

The first step in figuring out your next move is taking an inventory of how COPD is affecting your life. This can be more difficult, because many people have a hard time accepting even the limitations that age can put on them, much less the limitations of a chronic disease. You may be accustomed to "playing through the pain" and not letting mere physical ailments slow you down, for instance. But with COPD, pushing yourself the way you used to may be not only impractical — it may lead to worse symptoms or sudden attacks, which, in turn, can damage your overall health.

It's not easy to take an honest assessment of your limitations, so here are some questions to help you start thinking about how your COPD affects your life:

- ✔ Have you had to give up your job or switch to a part-time job because of your COPD?
- ✔ If you're still working, do you find that your job tires you out more than it used to?

✔ If you're still working, do you take more sick days than you used to?

✔ Have you given up or cut back on hobbies or activities that you used to look forward to?

✔ Does thinking about household chores (laundry, dusting, cooking, and so on) make you feel tired?

✔ Do you find socializing — either in person or on the phone — more tiring these days?

✔ Do you avoid certain activities because you're worried that you'll get too tired or that your symptoms will get worse?

Going over these questions with someone who knows you well may help. We all have blind spots, and an outside perspective sometimes can illuminate those areas.

Facing your fears

Fear is widely considered the most powerful of all human emotions. It's tied to a number of mental health issues, including development of anxiety disorders.

When you're told that you have COPD, or when you have a sudden attack of symptoms, your natural fears kick into overdrive. You may be scared by the very unpredictability of your COPD. You may be frightened because you feel you can't control your fate when you have COPD. You may fear becoming a burden on your family, being unable to care for yourself, and dying.

Talking about what scares you can deprive your fears of at least some of their power; it's like turning on the light for a child who thinks monsters are lurking in his closet. Your fears are normal, but you don't have to let them rule you.

COPD and sex

COPD can affect all aspects of your life, including your interest in, and ability to, engage in sexual activity. Talk with your doctor about your physical limitations when it comes to sex, how your medications may affect your ability to have sex, and mental and emotional issues that may interfere with your interest in sex. Talk with your spouse or partner, too. *Remember:* Sex isn't the only way to show your affection and maintain emotional intimacy with your partner. The most important thing is to be caring, loving, open, and honest with each other.

Grieving for your life as it used to be

We won't pretend that figuring out what you can't do (or don't want to do) anymore is a pleasant process. In fact, thinking in terms of what you *can't* do can be flat-out discouraging, if not depressing. Feeling a sense of loss and even getting angry about your limitations is normal. It's even normal to avoid thinking about your limitations so you don't have to deal with those feelings; for so many people, denial is a favorite coping mechanism.

It's okay to feel sorry for yourself. It's okay to grieve the loss of your physical health. It's okay to be frustrated and angry that you have this damned disease and ticked off at all the medications and doctors' appointments and tests and treatments involved in living with it. And it's okay to admit that you feel the way you do.

If you have a hard time figuring out how you feel, here are some techniques that may help:

- ✔ **Set a "grief appointment" with yourself.** Emotions don't always surface at convenient or appropriate times, but denying your emotions can make their effects worse. So instead of ignoring your feelings, make an appointment with yourself to deal with them. Set aside half an hour or an hour when you can be by yourself and allow yourself to feel what you're feeling. If it seems too self-indulgent, remember that feeling sorry for yourself is actually a way of comforting yourself. You may be surprised at how much better you feel after a good self-pity session.

- ✔ **Write down how you feel.** Many people aren't comfortable talking about how they feel, but they can release a lot of pent-up emotion in written form. What you write isn't for anyone's else eyes — unless you choose to share it — so you can be as brutally honest as you want.

- ✔ **Make a list of the challenges you've faced before COPD.** One of the reasons a diagnosis of COPD can be so devastating is because it's new and unknown — and it's normal to fear the unknown. But you've had to adjust to other challenges in your life, and remembering how you've dealt with those challenges can help build your confidence in dealing with your COPD.

- ✔ **Have a little ceremony to mark the passing of your old life.** All right, this sounds corny, and maybe it is. But sometimes a formal acknowledgement of your loss can help you face the future. The nice thing is that you decide how to honor your past life. And, by honoring your past life, you remind yourself of how you've met earlier challenges.

Getting adjusted to your new life

As you know from times when your life has changed in the past, getting used to a new routine takes some time. When you changed jobs or homes, when you had your first child or got your first pet, whenever you added a new wrinkle to your daily life, you had to learn how to adapt to accommodate the change. It's the same with COPD. No doubt you'll have a trial-and-error period before your everyday life runs like a well-oiled machine.

Patience is the key to making this adjustment as easy on yourself as possible. Don't expect everything to go perfectly right away, and don't beat yourself up when you forget part of your new routine or find that you don't have the energy to do everything you had hoped to do. Living with COPD involves a learning curve, and at first it'll feel foreign and uncomfortable. But that feeling will subside as you discover the tools, techniques, and patterns that work best for you.

Letting In Your Loved Ones

One of the most common reactions to a diagnosis of COPD — or any other serious health problem, for that matter — is a feeling of isolation. You're different now from the people around you; the label of a chronic illness erects an invisible barrier between you and everyone else.

The natural response to that feeling of being different is to ignore it. You put on a brave face; you're strong for your family; you reject others' attempts to express sympathy because you don't need it; you're careful never to complain about your condition.

The thing is, being strong and brave can add to your sense of isolation, because when you're always strong and brave, you don't let yourself show any weakness, either physically or emotionally. You can't ask for help if you're being strong, so you feel that you have to do everything on your own, which in turn makes you feel lonely, isolated, and even unloved. And various studies have shown that isolation and loneliness are harmful to both your mental health and your overall physical health.

It may not be easy to open up to your family and friends about the emotional effects of COPD. But you and they will feel better if you're all free to talk about the new reality and work out a sensible approach together.

Dealing with emotions

If you're like most people, you feel as though COPD has dumped you into a bizarre alternate universe, where nothing is what you thought it was or expected it to be and where you're buffeted by waves of confusing and conflicting emotions. You may feel overwhelmed by the lifestyle changes you have to make to manage your COPD. On days when your symptoms aren't bad, you may feel like it's all just a weird dream. On days when your symptoms keep you from doing what you normally do or what you want to do, you may feel the weight of discouragement. If you have a sudden flare-up, where your symptoms get rapidly worse, you may be just plain scared.

All these feelings are normal, and it's normal to have good and bad days both physically and emotionally. As you get accustomed to your new routine and begin doing the things you can do to manage your symptoms, these feelings may lose a lot of their initial force. That's not to say that you'll never experience their full impact again, but they may recede to the background for the most part.

There are some things you can do to keep bad feelings from taking over your life:

✔ **Get dressed every day, even if you don't plan to go out.** Motivating yourself to do something, even small household chores, is easier if you're already dressed and ready to face the day.

✔ **Whenever you can, take a walk outside for some exercise and fresh air.** Being cooped up isn't good for anybody's mental health. Even a few minutes outside can do wonders for your mood.

✔ **Keep up with favorite hobbies or activities, or, if that's not possible, find new ones.** Occupying your mind and hands with something you enjoy helps keep you from brooding about the not-so-positive things.

✔ **Maintain your friendships.** People are social creatures, and social interaction goes a long way in helping to keep your spirits up.

✔ **Talk to others — family members, friends, clergy, or a counselor — about how you feel.** Often, just expressing your feelings out loud can strip them of a lot of their force.

✔ **Take your meds as directed and follow the other elements of your treatment plan.** Your meds, diet, and exercise all play a role in reducing your physical symptoms, and the better you feel physically, the better you feel mentally and emotionally.

✔ **Give yourself permission to get enough rest.** COPD is a fatiguing disease, and if you don't get enough rest, you won't be able to do a lot of things you want to do.

Understanding resentment — on both sides

You're not the only one coping with a bewildering range of emotions. Your loved ones may take your COPD diagnosis on the chin mentally and emotionally, too. It's natural for them to be frightened and worried, to feel a sense of helplessness, and to be overwhelmed by the changes you and they must make to manage your condition well.

It's also natural for them — and for you — to feel angry and resentful. You're all mourning a loss. Just as you may feel bitter about not being able to do all the things you used to do, your family and friends may feel bitter that you aren't the same person who used to do so much with and for them.

It's not that they're blaming you for your illness, though it certainly can be misinterpreted that way. It's just that, after we form an impression of what kind of person our parent or spouse or sibling or friend is, it's very difficult to adjust that mental image to new realities. And part of the adjustment is a completely unreasonable and perfectly natural wish — often never spoken out loud — that things could go back to the way they used to be.

So this is what you've got: You and your loved ones both resent the limitations and changes that COPD forces on you. At the same time, both of you may be reluctant to express your feelings of frustration and anger; each of you may be trying to be as strong as you can for the other, thinking that will make it easier for the other to cope.

Believe it or not, acknowledging those feelings — and accepting that they're natural feelings to have on both sides — can do wonders to limit their potency. Frustration and resentment and all those other negative feelings are like mushrooms: They flourish when they're kept in the dark, but they find it harder to survive out in the open.

 Your family and friends may not want to bring up the emotional impact of your COPD for fear of upsetting or offending you. You can set the tone by starting the discussion yourself. Tell your loved ones how you're feeling, and ask them how they feel about your condition.

Figuring it out together

Like other challenges you and your family have faced, meeting the challenge of living well with COPD will take some teamwork. It may mean shifting responsibilities for household chores, or making different transportation arrangements, or even reorganizing one or more rooms of your home. Figuring out how to do these things together accomplishes two important goals: It gives your loved ones a constructive role in helping you manage your COPD, and it establishes a support system for you so you don't feel like you're facing this alone.

Much of the frustration your loved ones feel about your illness stems from a sense of powerlessness, a feeling of being unable to do anything to make it better. Involving them in planning and carrying out your new routine gives them a gratifying sense of being able to help.

Your family and friends can:

- ✔ **Help you stay active.** They can go for walks with you, take you shopping or to the hairdresser or to a movie, and accompany you to social activities.

- ✔ **Encourage you to follow your treatment plan.** They can help you make sure you're taking your meds correctly, eating properly, and getting enough rest and exercise.

- ✔ **Take over tasks that are too tiring for you.** They can take charge of grocery shopping, meal planning and cooking, housecleaning, and dozens of other chores and errands that you may find exhausting.

- ✔ **Provide emotional support.** They can lend a sympathetic ear when you need it, and a kick in the behind when you need that.

- ✔ **Protect your independence.** By helping out in all these ways, they allow you to remain as independent as possible for as long as possible.

Managing Stress

There's no question that COPD is a stressful disease, and stress can make the already wicked combination of its physical and emotional effects even more pronounced. It can be a vicious cycle: Your COPD makes you feel short of breath and fatigued; your physical symptoms make you feel anxious and worried; anxiety and worry make your breathing more rapid and shallow; rapid and shallow breathing makes you feel more short of breath; feeling more short of breath raises your anxiety level, which makes breathing even more difficult. . . . It's not a pretty picture — and it can even be dangerous, because this cycle can develop into a sudden worsening of your COPD symptoms, and sudden attacks can make your overall health get worse faster.

Knowing how to manage stress is critical to living well with COPD. Note that we didn't say "eliminate stress." That's impossible, even for the healthiest people; life is a stressful business. But, even though you can't make your life completely stress-free, you can use a variety of techniques to minimize its effects.

Relaxing the body and mind

Gentle stretches are effective at working tension out of muscles, and you can easily combine them with mental relaxation. When you feel your stress level building, take a few minutes to sit or lie quietly and focus on getting the tension out of your body. Start at either your head or your toes, and spend a few seconds concentrating on relaxing that part of your body. Then concentrate on doing the same thing with the next part of your body.

Controlled breathing is an excellent relaxation method. (Chapter 7 has illustrations and instructions for diaphragmatic and pursed-lip breathing.) To get the most benefit, exhale for twice as long as you inhale. This helps get more air out of your lungs and can reduce the sensation of being short of breath.

If you have trouble falling asleep, consciously relaxing each group of muscles can help. Start with your feet and work your way up, imagining the tension flowing out of your muscles at each step. By the time you reach your shoulders, you may find you're ready to sleep.

Audio tapes or CDs with relaxing music or other sounds can help you focus on mental and physical relaxation. There also are dozens of books and audio products filled with tips and techniques to promote relaxation. Start with *Meditation For Dummies,* 2nd Edition, by Stephan Bodian (Wiley) — it offers a CD with guided meditation exercises, as well as plenty of tips on bringing relaxation into all areas of your life.

Cutting back on stress inducers

One of the most common causes of stress is the feeling of being overloaded with responsibilities. When you have COPD, even mundane responsibilities like taking out the trash or washing the dishes can induce stress. Just as you have to learn to spend your physical energy wisely, you must decide what you want to spend your mental energy on, too.

This is where getting your family and friends involved comes in. With teamwork, you can delegate many responsibilities to others and leave yourself free to do the things that only you can do — like following your treatment and exercise program.

Taking care of yourself

Delegating responsibilities also leaves you free to take good care of yourself, and taking good care of yourself can add a lot of mileage to your stress-reduction efforts. Getting enough sleep and eating properly keep you physically prepared to handle the stress you can't avoid. Exercise, a critical component of your COPD management plan, is an excellent stress-reliever in itself.

Finding Other Support

Friends, clergy, and counselors can help you work through those times when you feel you just don't have the strength to do it on your own. Pouring your troubles and worries into a sympathetic ear relieves much of the emotional and mental burden you carry, and sometimes just talking things over with someone outside your immediate family can present options and perspectives you wouldn't have thought of otherwise.

Support from others also is a key part of warding off loneliness and feelings of isolation, both of which can make your physical health worse.

People like you: COPD groups

People who aren't familiar with COPD may not fully understand the challenges you face, and suggestions for making your life easier may not be practical or appropriate for you. You may find that a COPD support group can provide just that extra fillip of personal experience and understanding that you need.

Ask your doctor if there's a COPD group in your area. Your local library or social service agency may be able to help you find one, too. And, of course, there's always the Internet; there are thousands of sites with information about COPD and dozens of online communities for COPD patients and their families. (See Chapter 20 for some Web sites to get you started.)

Talking it out: What therapy can do

If you can't seem to shake negative feelings and those feelings interfere with your ability to cope with your COPD and find ways to enjoy life, you may want to consider professional counseling. Persistent feelings of helplessness, worthlessness, and sorrow can indicate depression, which can seriously hinder your efforts to manage the physical effects of COPD.

The National Institute of Mental Health cites these additional indicators for depression that should be evaluated and treated by a counselor or psychiatrist:

- ✔ Pessimism
- ✔ Guilt

- ✔ Loss of interest in hobbies and other activities
- ✔ Low energy levels
- ✔ Changes in sleep patterns (insomnia or excessive sleeping)
- ✔ Changes in appetite or weight
- ✔ Restlessness
- ✔ Tension or irritability
- ✔ Difficulty with concentration or making decisions
- ✔ Thoughts of suicide or death

Notice that some symptoms of depression — low energy levels, changes in weight or appetite, difficulty concentrating — are also effects of COPD. You may have trouble knowing whether your symptoms are physical, emotional, or a combination of the two.

Depression is more than just a passing bad mood or case of the blahs. Research shows that depression can do more damage to your physical health than many chronic diseases, including arthritis, diabetes, asthma, and some forms of heart disease. When you have depression in addition to a chronic disease, it makes your chronic disease worse; researchers found that living for one year with both diabetes and depression puts you at just 60 percent of full health.

An effective COPD treatment plan is comprehensive, covering both your physical and mental health. Ask your doctor about including counseling in your treatment plan. Also ask about free or sliding-fee mental health services that may be appropriate.

Before you go to a counselor, check your health insurance policy for coverage restrictions on mental health services. Some plans will pay for it, some will pay a portion, and some either don't cover it at all or approve it only under certain circumstances.

Considering antidepressants

Antidepressants have come a long way over the last several decades, but perceptions and stigmas are slow to change. For many people, the term *antidepressant* conjures up visions of zombie-like people who are too high-strung or otherwise mentally "weak" to deal with the rough and tumble of real life. These kinds of persistent stereotypes and misconceptions may explain why, in one study of the effect of antidepressants on COPD patients, a majority of patients who were diagnosed with depression refused antidepressant therapy.

So let's talk about what you can really expect from today's antidepressants. They won't get you high, nor will they turn you into some vacant-eyed horror-show creature. Newer drugs work by correcting an imbalance in brain chemicals, so you feel more like yourself mentally and emotionally. Some people describe their antidepressant medication as "taking the edge off" their feelings of anxiety, panic, and depression.

Of course, like any medication, antidepressants can cause unwanted side effects. Some antidepressants make it harder for you to lose weight and may actually promote weight gain; depending on your situation, this may not be a concern for you or your doctor. Some of them may interfere with your sleep patterns, causing insomnia or vivid, even bizarre, dreams; some can make you feel tired or drowsy during the day. Some can upset your stomach unless you eat something right before or right after you take them. Some may lower your sex drive, but, if depression has been inhibiting your sex drive, you may find your interest in sex is higher after you start taking an antidepressant.

Antidepressants, like other prescription drugs, can interfere with some medications. Talk to your doctor about the pros and cons of antidepressants and how they may interact with your other meds.

If you're trying to quit smoking, an antidepressant can help ease the nervousness and irritability that often accompanies nicotine withdrawal. One of the most commonly prescribed stop-smoking aids, in fact, is called Wellbutrin when it's prescribed as an antidepressant but named Zyban when it's prescribed as a stop-smoking aid.

Developing Coping Strategies

COPD is one of those conditions that produces highly individualized symptoms, and the right strategies to cope well with your COPD may not be the same strategies that work for someone else. As you become more familiar with COPD and how it affects you and your lifestyle, you'll find some tips and techniques offered by others that work beautifully and some that don't quite fit your needs.

Here are some steps that can help you develop your own coping strategies:

- ✔ **Research COPD.** Knowledge is power, and the more you know about COPD and how it's affecting you, the better prepared you are to adapt to your changing needs.
- ✔ **See your doctor every six months.** Regular appointments are the easiest way to monitor the progress of your COPD and your general health.

✔ **Know how to use your meds.** If you don't use your medications properly, you can't manage your COPD symptoms as well. If the instructions are confusing, ask your doctor or pharmacist for clarification.

✔ **Follow your exercise and diet plans.** Staying fit and making sure you get the proper nutrition can do a lot to keep your COPD symptoms under control.

✔ **Find ways to enjoy life.** Even if you can't do some of the things you used to, there are still things you can enjoy. Learning new skills and exploring new activities help keep your mind sharp and your spirits up.

Chapter 6

Building Your Healthcare Team

*T*here's a popular misconception that, because COPD can't be cured, it can't be treated. There is a difference between curing a disease and managing it, and when it comes to COPD, managing the disease well means managing virtually every aspect of your physical and mental health.

Your healthcare team can help you do just that. It starts with your primary-care physician, who is familiar with your overall health and can provide you with information, tests, and checkups to make sure other potential health concerns don't get forgotten in the efforts to treat your COPD symptoms.

Your primary-care physician also is an invaluable contact for referrals to specialists and programs that can help you with your COPD. Specialists may include a pulmonologist, who has additional training and expertise in treating lung disease; a nutritionist or registered dietitian, who can help you design a healthy eating plan that suits your needs and lifestyle; an occupational therapist, who can show you ways to adjust your routine and the way you move your body to conserve energy; and perhaps a counselor or therapist, who can help you cope with the common emotional and mental aspects of being diagnosed with a chronic disease.

In this chapter, we introduce you to each of these potential members of your healthcare team. We tell you what each of them does and how what they do fits in with treating your COPD. We show you what to look for in choosing your healthcare team, give you some questions to ask during your search, and offer tips on where to find the information you need.

And, just in case you don't yet have a doctor you see regularly, we start off with a quick guide to finding the right primary-care doctor for you.

Finding a Doctor

There are lots of reasons why you may not have a doctor at the moment. Maybe your doctor retired recently and you haven't gotten around to finding another one. Maybe you don't really like the doctor you used to see, and rather than just move on to another one, you've avoided doctors altogether. Maybe you've moved or changed jobs or insurance plans. Maybe you've been basically healthy for so many years that you just never felt the need to establish a long-term relationship with a specific doctor.

But when you have COPD, or suspect you may have it, it's time to get serious about finding a doctor you're comfortable with. For one thing, your health insurer may not pay for the care of a specialist unless your primary-care physician first makes a referral. For another, even if you've never gone in for regular checkups before, you're going to have to build them into your schedule now, and regular checkups are a lot more useful — and a lot less hassle — if the same doctor sees you each time.

What kind of doctor do you want?

Your primary-care doctor — what most people call their "regular" doctor — likely will be a family practitioner, an internist, a geriatrician, or perhaps an osteopath. All these types of doctors can diagnose and treat a broad spectrum of health conditions; they order tests like blood work and X-rays; and they provide referrals to specialists when necessary.

Here's how these primary-care doctors differ:

- **Family practitioners:** These doctors get training in healthcare for all members of a family, from infants to the elderly, and also in the treatment of pregnant women.

- **Internists:** Internists generally treat adult patients only.

- **Geriatricians:** These are doctors who've taken additional training in treating aging and elderly patients.

- **Osteopaths:** These healthcare providers use the designation DO after their names; they tend to take a more holistic approach to medicine, incorporating physical, mental, and emotional factors into their diagnoses and treatments. Like MDs, some DOs specialize in certain areas of medicine, but some are primary-care physicians, too.

For the sake of convenience, we use the terms *doctor* and *physician* here. But your primary healthcare professional doesn't necessarily have to have the letters *MD* after his name. Physician's assistants and nurse practitioners, who work under the supervision of an MD and who have to meet strict continuing education requirements to keep their certifications, often are able to spend more time with patients on office visits than physicians are.

No matter which kind of doctor you choose, you want one who will provide the treatment you need when you need it. You want to make sure you're getting the right kinds of tests and medications, that you're not being subjected to tests or procedures you don't need, and that you're not being put at risk through dangerous combinations of medications (see the "What to look for" section later in this chapter).

Where to look

You could grab the nearest phone book and start making cold calls to doctors in your area. But most people are more comfortable getting a recommendation from a family member or friends. You can ask them what they like about their doctor, what their experience has been in scheduling appointments and tests, and how the doctor's office handles insurance claims.

If you need to look further, try contacting a nearby hospital or your local medical society. If there's a medical school in your area, check to see if it has a referral service for new patients. You can also check the phone book for a local physician's referral service.

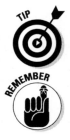

If you're looking for a new doctor because your old doctor is retiring or moving out of the area, ask your old doctor if she can recommend a new doctor for you. Also ask about transferring your medical records to your new doctor.

When you're shopping for a doctor, there are two critical questions to ask before you even make your first appointment:

✔ Is the doctor accepting new patients?

✔ Does the doctor accept your health insurance?

A no to either of these questions means you need to continue your search.

What to look for

When you have a list of doctors who are accepting new patients and who participate in your health insurance plan, you can start narrowing the field by adding other criteria. Some things that may influence your decision:

- ✔ **Convenience:** How difficult would it be for you to get to the doctor's office? Does the office have enough parking? Is parking free? Does the doctor offer evening or weekend appointments so you don't have to take time off work? Is there a lab on-site to conduct routine blood tests and X-rays? Is there a pharmacy on-site or nearby?

- ✔ **Training and experience:** Does the doctor have extra training for his practice, such as board certification in internal medicine or family practice? How long has the doctor been in practice? Does she see many patients with health issues similar to yours?

- ✔ **Affiliations:** Which hospital is the doctor affiliated with? Would you be comfortable being treated at that hospital if necessary? Which specialists does the doctor usually recommend for people with your health conditions? Does the doctor have a particular lab or pharmacy of choice if there isn't one on site? Where are the lab and pharmacy located, and how easy will it be for you to get there?

- ✔ **Office operations:** How does the doctor's office handle insurance claims? If the doctor is unavailable to see patients, who covers for him? Can you get in to see the doctor immediately if necessary? Does the office call patients to remind them of appointments, tests, prescription refills, and so on?

- ✔ **Reputation:** Word of mouth can tell you much about whether a specific doctor or clinic may be right for you. You also may be able to find report cards or quality reports about doctors and hospitals in your area. Some of these may include consumer reviews, and some may include reviews by governmental agencies. For instance, the U.S. Department of Health and Human Services offers an online tool to compare hospitals and the care they provide; you can check out hospitals in your area at www. hospitalcompare.hhs.gov.

 Your employer or health insurance plan may have quality reports available for local healthcare providers. You also can call hospitals and clinics directly and ask if they have quality reports available. If you need more help, contact your local library or state health department.

The comfort factor

When it comes right down to it, the most experienced doctor with the best reputation in the most convenient location will be no good to you at all if you don't feel comfortable with her. It's no accident that we called this chapter

"Building Your Healthcare *Team*." You and your doctor have to be able to work together to address your health. You need a doctor you can look on as a partner, a teammate in managing your health.

Communication and rapport are critical elements in a good doctor-patient relationship. In fact, studies have shown that the better you understand what your doctor is talking about, the healthier and longer-lived you can expect to be. If you don't understand what your doctor tells you, the research indicates, you're less likely to take your prescriptions properly, less likely to make preventive or wellness visits to your doctor, less likely to properly manage chronic diseases (COPD, high blood pressure, diabetes, and so on), and more likely to end up in the emergency room or hospital.

Here are some signs that it may be time to find a different doctor:

✔ Your doctor doesn't listen to your concerns about medications or treatment options and insists you do things his way.

✔ Your doctor doesn't like it when you ask questions.

✔ Your doctor seems rushed, impatient, or distracted during your visits.

✔ You leave your doctor's office feeling stressed, tired, or otherwise bad about the visit.

✔ You start putting off visits to your doctor because you anticipate a bad experience.

Sometimes personality or philosophy conflicts occur between doctors and patients, too. Don't feel guilty if you just don't like a particular doctor, or if you sense that the doctor doesn't like you. The doctor-patient relationship is like any other; it's more difficult to work together if you don't particularly care for each other's style. Save yourself (and the doctor) time and energy and find a doctor you can work with.

First Stop: Your Primary-Care Physician

Think of your primary-care physician as your default for all the medical care you need. She should be your first stop not only for regular checkups, but whenever a problem arises. Your regular doctor knows your medical history and, perhaps most important, knows how to interpret various signs and symptoms of disease and recommend appropriate treatments or referrals.

Why is this so important? Because all that wheezes is not COPD, or even a lung issue. In fact, difficulty breathing is more likely an indicator of heart problems than of lung disease. Conditions like anemia also can cause breathing difficulties. And going to a pulmonologist when you have cardiac problems or iron-deficiency anemia is a waste of time and money.

Assessing your general health

Your regular doctor can determine whether your shortness of breath is really a lung problem or something else, and he can refer you to the proper specialists if necessary. Just as important, though, your regular doctor is focused on maintaining your overall wellness, not just on treating health problems. So you can turn to your regular doctor for advice on exercise, nutrition, and a myriad of other topics.

COPD is often complicated by other chronic conditions like high blood pressure, obesity, diabetes, or arthritis. It's critical to keep track of treatments for all these things to make sure your prescriptions don't interfere with each other or produce alarming side effects.

Your regular doctor also can provide you with preventive care like flu shots and pneumonia vaccine — both highly recommended for COPD patients.

Tracking vital functions

Regular checkups allow your doctor to keep track of things like your blood pressure, pulse, and breathing rate. She gets a good idea of what's normal for you for each of these functions, and, therefore, is better equipped to decide when changes in your normal readings merit further investigation. Some cold medications can raise your blood pressure, for example, so your regular doctor probably won't be too concerned if your blood pressure is higher than normal when you tell her you're taking something for your cold. On the other hand, if your blood pressure is higher than normal and there's no clear explanation for it, that alerts your doctor to keep a close eye on it to see if it requires treatment.

Getting referrals to specialists

Some health insurance plans won't cover visits to specialists unless your primary doctor makes a referral. This is because insurers want to make sure the (typically) higher costs associated with referrals are justified; the primary doctor acts as a screener, deciding who he can treat and who needs the services of a specialist.

There are other benefits to using your primary doctor as a referral service. Chances are your doctor is familiar with the specialist's qualifications, treatment philosophy and interaction with patients, and ability to effectively treat you; you don't have to go through the same "shopping" process for specialists that you used to find your primary doctor. And, as a matter of convenience, your primary doctor and specialist usually will share your medical records and reports with each other, so each of them knows what the other is doing.

Answering your questions

Your primary doctor is an encyclopedia of knowledge. More than likely, she can answer nearly any question you may have about your condition and your treatment, including how and why certain tests may be performed, common side effects of medications, and tips on improving or maintaining your overall health. Most doctors' offices have brochures or other literature that you can take home and review at your leisure, and most of them can refer you to outside sources of information, like Web sites or support groups.

The Pulmonologist

Pulmonologists are doctors who specialize in lung disease. They have to be board-certified in internal medicine before they can pursue additional training and certification in pulmonology. This training includes graduate instruction on the structure and function of the lungs, how the immune system protects and affects the lungs, and various lung diseases, as well as training in diagnosing and managing lung problems. Most pulmonologists also are trained in critical care, including various methods of mechanical ventilation — what most people think of as "life support." Pulmonologists can care for patients in every stage of COPD, from the person with mild COPD who only needs office visits every six months to the one with advanced-stage COPD in need of mechanical breathing assistance.

What a pulmonologist looks for

The pulmonologist is interested in how well you breathe in and out and how much oxygen your body manages to get into your blood stream. For COPD patients, the real problem is getting air *out* of the lungs. Air tends to get trapped in the bottom of your lungs because you can't exhale fully, and this, in turn, makes it difficult to inhale. This is the cycle that makes you feel like you can't catch your breath.

Your primary doctor may conduct a spirometry test to measure your lungs' air capacity. Two essential components of spirometry are *forced expiratory volume in the first second* (FEV1), which measures how much air you can force out of your lungs in 1 second, and *forced vital capacity* (FVC), which measures how much air you can exhale period, with no time limit. If you go to a pulmonologist without seeing your primary doctor first, the pulmonologist will order the spirometry test.

Your pulmonologist also may order or administer more sophisticated tests that confirm the COPD diagnosis and give him much more information to evaluate the severity of the disease. In addition, he may order tests that show

how much oxygen your blood carries, chest X-rays and *echocardiograms* (ultrasounds of your heart), and even *bronchoscopy* (a minimally invasive medical procedure that allows the pulmonologist to look inside your bronchial tubes and, if necessary, remove fluid or tissue).

Your pulmonologist probably will ask you things like how far you walk before stopping, if you have trouble breathing when you go up a flight of stairs, and so on. But the way the questions are phrased may not lead to the whole story, so be sure to add any details that are relevant. For example, if the longest distance you ever walk is 2 blocks to the grocery store, or if the longest flight of stairs you typically encounter is only four or five steps, that may not be a good indication of your true abilities or limitations.

How a pulmonologist can help

After assessing the results of your tests, your pulmonologist will prescribe medications and may recommend certain devices that help you breathe — metered dose inhalers and nebulizers, for example. (See Chapter 8 for information on treatment options.) Depending on the severity of your COPD and other health conditions, she may refer you to other specialists, such as a dietitian or occupational therapist (we discuss their roles in the following section), and she may even recommend a pulmonary rehabilitation program for you, which is a combination of medical treatment, exercise, nutrition, and counseling.

Many insurance plans won't approve the use of things like breathing machines and oxygen delivery systems unless certain tests have been performed and show the devices are needed. This is another area in which seeing a pulmonologist can help; she knows what tests to conduct to determine the best treatment options.

The Dietitian or Nutritionist

Eating properly is a critical component of managing your COPD, so your primary doctor or pulmonologist may recommend that you see a dietitian or nutritionist to work out a healthy diet plan. These people can show you what a balanced diet looks like, provide tips on getting more healthy foods into your diet, and even plan out menus for you to follow.

Although many people use the terms *dietitian* and *nutritionist* interchangeably, there are differences — mainly in the level of training and education — between the two. A registered dietitian must have a bachelor's degree and complete an internship and other training before qualifying for the RD credential. Registered dietitians sometimes call themselves nutritionists because that term is more recognizable for many people; the *nutritionist* label also may be less intimidating, because many people shy away from the concept of "dieting" but are interested in how food can affect their health.

There is no uniform definition for the term *nutritionist,* so the level of education and training can vary widely. Those who are licensed nutritionists, certified clinical nutritionists, or certified nutrition specialists must have at least a bachelor's degree in nutrition, food science, or a related field.

Improved nutrition equals better health

The better you eat, the better your overall health. That's true for everybody, and it's especially important when you have COPD, because you need every bit of help you can get in maintaining your current lung function and fighting off infections and other complications. Certain conditions like anemia can affect the ability of your blood to transport oxygen throughout your body, for example, and low levels of electrolytes like phosphorus can hinder pulmonary performance because respiratory muscles become weaker.

Dietitians and nutritionists who work with COPD patients understand the unique goals and challenges those patients face in establishing healthy eating patterns. (We devote Chapter 11 to the particular nutritional needs of COPD patients.) Their goal in working with you will be to help you get the nutrition you need from meals and, if necessary, supplements.

Assessing your eating habits

The dietitian or nutritionist will want to know about your eating habits now so he can figure out what changes may be necessary. Being honest is important; if you have a sweet tooth or a fondness for salty snacks, don't let guilt keep you from telling him about your afternoon chocolate bar or the chips and dip you like to munch on while watching TV.

Talking about any obstacles you face in trying to eat better is also important. Maybe your appetite has waned and you just don't feel like eating most of the time. Maybe you find it too tiring to plan and prepare honest-to-goodness meals, so you fall back on prepackaged convenience foods. Maybe cost is an issue; after all, milk, meats, fruits, and vegetables are expensive, and the cost seems to be going up all the time. Your dietitian or nutritionist needs to know about all these things so he can figure out the best way to help you.

Setting nutritional goals

Together, you and your dietitian should decide what you'd like to accomplish with a better diet. Because weight control — either losing weight or maintaining a healthy weight — is so important for COPD patients (see Chapter 11), this will be one of the main goals of your eating plan. Other goals may include feeling more energetic, controlling high blood pressure and/or cholesterol, or managing diabetes.

Your dietitian can explain how your eating plan can help you accomplish your goals and offer tips to help you stay on track. And when you know what you want to accomplish, the two of you can work out a sensible plan to get there.

Creating a regimen that works for you

Once your dietitian has the information she needs, the next step is to create an eating plan that makes sense for you. This plan should take into account not only your COPD, but any other health issues you may have, such as high blood pressure or diabetes. It should reflect the way you eat — whether you prefer three regular meals a day with no snacks or a series of more than three smaller meals spread out throughout the day.

Ideally, your eating plan should incorporate plenty of foods you like. Sticking to a regimen is almost impossible if you don't like most of what it includes, so be honest with your dietitian about what you do and don't like to eat. If you can't stand bananas, for example, your dietitian can recommend other foods that will provide you with the potassium and other nutrients found in bananas. Your dietitian also may have tips and tricks for sneaking foods you should have (but don't like to eat) into dishes you do like.

And finally, your eating plan should reflect any challenges or obstacles in your situation. If you can't afford to buy fresh fruits and vegetables every week, your dietitian should be able to recommend lower-cost alternatives. If you have trouble working up the energy to cook, your dietitian should be able to show you how to make healthier choices when you shop for already-prepared foods.

The Occupational Therapist

The term *occupational therapy* can be misleading because it seems to imply work-related activities. In fact, occupational therapy is designed to help you work around whatever physical limitations you may have. For COPD patients, the focus is often on the home: learning ways to make routine tasks easier for you and less tiring. The ultimate goal of occupational therapy is to allow you to remain independent as long as possible.

Every state licenses or otherwise regulates occupational therapists. Beginning in 2007, they must have at least a master's degree from an accredited educational program (the previous minimum was a bachelor's degree), and they have to pass a national certification test. When they meet those criteria, they're allowed to use the title *occupational therapist registered* (OTR).

Your therapy may actually be conducted by an occupational therapy assistant. They work under the supervision of an OTR and are required to have an associate's degree or a certificate from an accredited technical program.

Occupational therapist *aides* are not the same as occupational therapy *assistants*. Whereas assistants conduct therapy sessions with clients, aides generally provide clerical assistance to OTRs, and most of their training is on-the-job. When you enroll in an occupational therapy program, be sure to ask about the education and training of the people you'll be working with.

Helping you achieve your daily goals

In general, occupational therapy is concerned with *general life skills* — the abilities that allow you to function independently, from personal hygiene to budgeting to shopping to cooking. For COPD patients, therapy also focuses on saving energy and getting the most out your breathing ability. So your therapist may show you how to reorganize your kitchen to be more convenient and efficient, or suggest devices like safety rails next to the toilet or tub. If you need to use a wheelchair or motorized scooter to get around, he may show you how to maneuver it and make changes in your home to accommodate it.

You can make occupational therapy more effective by figuring out what you'd like to be able to do every day and asking your therapist to help you devise comfortable and convenient ways to accomplish those goals. Here are some areas where your therapist may be able to help:

- ✔ **Mobility:** If you have trouble getting around, either at home or when you're out, ask your therapist for ideas to make it easier. If you want to avoid or delay using devices like a walker or wheelchair, your therapist can recommend exercises and strategies that will help maintain your ability to walk on your own.

- ✔ **Self-care:** Bathing, dressing, and grooming can be a challenge, if not exhausting, when you have COPD. Your occupational therapist can show you energy-saving techniques and recommend things like shower chairs or safety mats.

✔ **Socializing:** Feeling isolated from friends and even family is a big issue for people with chronic diseases, and COPD is no exception. Your therapist can help you arrange your home so you can be comfortable and still be involved in social activities.

If your doctor or pulmonologist doesn't recommend occupational therapy, ask about getting a consultation — including a home inspection and evaluation — anyway. Even if your COPD is only mild or moderate, an occupational therapist can recommend changes around your home that will help you stay independent longer.

Targeted exercise for your goals

COPD often is associated with muscle weakness, especially in the upper body and in the legs. Targeted exercise can help preserve and improve muscle strength, which, in turn, enables you to do more and to remain independent longer. Your occupational therapist will show you how to do certain exercises and explain how they help.

Upper-body strength

Your body uses more energy — and puts a higher demand on your lungs — when you use your arms, shoulders, chest, and neck. This is why some daily activities, like bathing, dressing, and grooming, can be so tiring when you have COPD. It's also why carrying things like groceries and laundry baskets can be difficult, and why you may feel nervous about pulling heavy objects from upper shelves in the kitchen or closet.

Upper-body exercises typically are designed to improve flexibility, strength, and range of motion. Your therapist may have you place a long, wide band of rubber under your feet and pull up with both hands, for instance, to strengthen both your grip and the muscles in your arms and shoulders.

The goal of any exercise program is to increase your tolerance for and ability to move around. Even if you have the strength to do your exercises for only a couple of minutes each day, investing those couple of minutes is important. A regular exercise routine will help you keep whatever strength you've got and, eventually, make you stronger.

Lower-body strength

Weakness in the legs is common with COPD, and that's not surprising. After all, if you have trouble breathing, you're not likely to increase your activity level, and the lack of activity leads to loss of muscle tone and mass. Then, when you do try to increase your activity level, you find yourself fighting harder for breath at even lower levels of exertion, and you feel so weak that you can't do much anyway.

Research indicates that COPD patients benefit more from an exercise program that includes specific arm and leg exercises than from a generic program. Breathing capacity and quality of life both are higher in people with COPD who use a targeted exercise program.

Treadmill walking and stationary cycling are often recommended for COPD patients, but make sure you're ready and able to undergo this type of exercise. If your COPD symptoms don't seem to be well-controlled, talk to your doctor before starting any exercise program.

The Counselor

According to a Canadian study, close to half of all COPD patients also suffer from depression, anxiety, or other mental health issues. That compares with less than a third of the general population, which means just being diagnosed with COPD puts you at higher risk for psychiatric problems. If you're a woman with COPD, you're also more likely than your male counterpart to suffer from at least one mental health problem, and more likely to have an anxiety disorder, panic disorder, or a phobia. (We talk about the emotional impact of COPD in detail in Chapter 5.)

Feelings of powerlessness and hopelessness are nothing unusual when you have COPD, but they can be difficult to overcome on your own. Very often, these feelings stem from the fear of an acute attack (see Chapter 16), and it becomes a vicious downward cycle, both physically and psychologically.

There may be other things going on, too, that are causing stress, depression, and anxiety. A licensed counselor can help you identify and work through the psychological aspects of living with COPD.

Licensed mental health counselors must have at least a master's degree in counseling or a related mental health field and must have at least two years of experience working as a counselor under the supervision of a licensed counselor, psychologist, or psychiatrist. Counselors also have to pass state exams to receive their licenses.

Licensed counselors charge less than psychologists or psychiatrists, and most insurance plans that cover mental health expenses will cover sessions with licensed counselors. Check with your insurance plan to find out your coverage requirements and limitations.

Many counselors offer sliding-scale fees for clients based on income. If cost is a concern, ask your doctor to recommend a counselor who can accommodate your budget.

Dealing with depression

Depression is more common than you may think, and it's especially common among COPD sufferers — even more especially among women with COPD. Counseling and, sometimes (depending on what other medications you're taking), antidepressants can alleviate the effects of depression.

Identifying and addressing depression is important because, according to recent research, depression does more damage to your overall health than chronic disease does. Researchers looked at World Health Organization data from 60 countries and found that when depression is combined with a chronic disease, the effects of the actual disease are worse. If you go for a year with a chronic illness and depression, your overall health is reduced by 40 percent. People with depression also report more problems with mobility, memory, and vision, the research showed.

Ignoring your symptoms of depression won't make them go away, and depression severely limits your ability to manage your COPD. If you think you may suffer from depression, talk to your primary doctor; she can recommend a counselor and perhaps medication to help you deal with it.

Some signs to look for:

- ✔ You lose interest in hobbies or activities that you used to enjoy.
- ✔ You can't seem to shake feelings of sadness or anxiety.
- ✔ You have a hard time sleeping, or you sleep more than you need to.
- ✔ Your appetite or weight has changed (up or down) for no apparent reason.
- ✔ You have a hard time concentrating or have difficulty making decisions.

A comprehensive program that includes exercise, education, physical therapy, and breathing and relaxation exercises can be just as effective, if not more effective, in countering anxiety and depression than counseling alone. This is probably because physical and psychological conditions are so closely intertwined; it makes sense that results are better when you take an inclusive approach to treatment and therapy.

Keeping up your mental energy

Just as depression can put you in a cycle of ever-worsening health and declining energy, a positive outlook can help you manage your COPD better, and perhaps even slow its progress.

Mounting research shows that a positive mental outlook has definite health benefits. Optimists have stronger immune systems and recover more quickly from illness, injury, and surgery. When it comes to chronic illnesses like COPD, they tend to have less severe symptoms and less frequent acute attacks.

So how do you cultivate a positive mental outlook? Here are some things that can help you feel more cheerful and upbeat:

✔ **Exercise.** Part of the reason your doctor wants you to exercise, even if only a tiny bit, is because exercise does wonders for your mental health. (We discuss the advantages of exercise in detail in Chapter 12.) Movement stimulates the natural feel-good chemicals in your brain, and the more of those feel-good chemicals you can release, the less severe your physical symptoms seem.

✔ **Keep up your social connections.** Isolation and loneliness, especially among the elderly, can be just as debilitating as physical ailments. Make an effort to keep in touch with friends and family. If you can't go out on the town like you used to, ask people to visit you in your home. Use the telephone and e-mail to stay connected with the people who mean the most to you.

✔ **Count your blessings.** It sounds trite and corny, but research has shown that people who focus on the good things in their lives feel happier and more satisfied. You can use several techniques to remind yourself of the things that make life good for you. You can try keeping a gratitude journal, in which you write down events and things that you're grateful for or that make you feel happy. Or, before you go to sleep each night, think of three good things that happened that day; if you can think of more than three, even better.

Balancing wild hopes and realistic expectations

Of course, we're not suggesting that you adopt a Pollyanna attitude toward life or your illness. In psychiatric terms, that kind of unrealistic optimism is called *denial,* and it won't help you do what really is necessary to manage your COPD.

Your doctor and other members of your healthcare team can help you take a realistic approach to dealing with your condition. Listen to them and to your own body; you'll find it's fairly easy to figure out what's possible now; what you can accomplish with medications, diet, and exercise; and what is most likely beyond human control.

Being realistic isn't the same as being pessimistic. Pessimists expect the worst. Realists know the difference between the possible and the unlikely, and they focus their attention on what's possible. It's a reasonable balance, because overblown expectations inevitably lead to disappointment, and repeated disappointments can spark depression. When you're realistic about your condition, your limitations, and your goals, you set yourself up for success instead of failure.

Pulmonary Rehabilitation

Pulmonary rehabilitation is really just a fancy term for a program that includes many of the things we cover in earlier portions of this chapter. A formal program combines education about COPD, medical treatment, exercise, counseling, and nutrition advice. Much of the program is usually carried out at a clinic or rehab center, which provides a safe and supervised environment for exercising and counseling.

Rehab goals

The goals of any pulmonary rehab program are to control and ease the symptoms of COPD and, therefore, to improve the patient's quality of life — and maybe even extend the patient's life expectancy. Research indicates that the multidisciplinary approach does a pretty good job of attaining those goals, too. Patients who take part in rehab improve their tolerance for movement and activity and are able to engage in movement and activity for longer periods. They also report fewer episodes of feeling short of breath and a better quality of life. Finally, and significantly, rehab reduces healthcare costs because those patients typically don't use emergency and hospital services as much as COPD patients who aren't in a rehab program.

There's no evidence that your lung function actually improves with pulmonary rehabilitation when you have COPD. However, it does help you maximize your existing lung function, and the other health benefits of exercise, nutrition, and counseling help make breathing easier and improve your quality of life.

A formal rehab program may include exercises and therapies that you wouldn't otherwise use, and some that you may already be using. For example, most pulmonary rehab programs include training in controlled breathing techniques such as diaphragmatic breathing or pursed-lip breathing (you can find illustrations of these techniques in Chapter 7). But you're likely already using one or more of these breathing techniques; COPD patients seem to instinctively find the method that works for them to ease their symptoms.

Other techniques do require training if you're to do them properly and without risking injury. Techniques like *postural drainage* and *chest percussion* are effective ways to clear the airways of mucus, but, to be safe and effective, you need specific instructions from a rehab specialist who is familiar with the technique. And, until you're completely comfortable with it, you shouldn't use these techniques except under the supervision of your rehab specialist.

Who needs rehab

Many doctors and pulmonologists routinely recommend rehab only for their patients with severe, late-stage COPD. Research shows that even patients who are so sick that they need lung surgery or a transplant can improve their overall fitness and lung function with the proper rehab program.

There's also a growing body of evidence that early rehab can at least delay and perhaps even prevent the progress of COPD. Like most diseases, the earlier COPD is diagnosed and properly treated, the less likely it is to cause serious disruptions in your life. And, of course, the less severe the disease, the lower the costs — in time, money, and energy — of treating it effectively.

Even if your COPD is in the mild or moderate stage, ask your doctor about pulmonary rehab. If your doctor seems reluctant to recommend it for you, ask him if it makes sense as a preventive measure — a way to help slow the progress of your COPD.

The key to a successful rehab program is an individualized structure. Every element of your rehab program should be geared toward your specific needs, from your tolerance for certain forms of exercise to your diet to your goals for everyday living.

Chapter 7

COPD Treatment Goals

*T*here is no cure for COPD, so treatment generally focuses on slowing down the progress of the disease and managing your symptoms. The goal is to keep you as healthy as possible, prevent complications, and minimize the severity of your symptoms so you can still enjoy your life.

Developing a treatment plan that works best for you can be a lengthy process; it make take several weeks or even several months. Even after you've got a treatment plan that controls your symptoms, you may have to tweak it every now and then. The time of year, weather conditions, your activity level, and dozens of other variables can affect how well your treatment plan works at any given moment. Even the aging process can trigger changes in how your body responds to various medications, so doses may need to be changed or you may need to switch to different drugs.

This is why it's so important that you feel comfortable with and confident in your doctor. Each of you has vital responsibilities in meeting the goals you set, and because the best way to achieve your goals may change, you need to be able to communicate well with each other.

In this chapter, we take you through the realistic goals you and your doctor should have about controlling your COPD. Your first priority is to control your symptoms and slow the progress of the disease. Your doctor can prescribe medications to help with this, but your lifestyle choices are just as important, so in this chapter we discuss both. Avoiding complications when possible and treating those that arise is the next step; we walk you through some of the common problems COPD patients have to deal with, including other health problems and sudden attacks of severe COPD symptoms. Finally, we cover the importance of preserving your existing lung function for as long as possible.

Controlling Progression and Symptoms

The earlier that COPD is diagnosed, the easier it is to manage and the less it affects your overall health and quality of life. But even if you have moderate or severe COPD, your treatment program will be designed to slow down the progression of your illness as much as possible. Your doctor also will want to lower both the frequency and the severity of sudden attacks, because these can do serious damage to your overall health.

Changing your lifestyle to ease symptoms

Much of what your doctor tells you to do won't seem like medicine at all: Quit smoking, eat better, lose (or gain) weight, and exercise. We talk about each of these things in detail in Part III. Here, we want to stress the importance of lifestyle changes on your overall health.

Quitting smoking

No matter how far along your COPD is, quitting smoking is your first defense against causing more damage. Some patients figure there's no reason to quit after they've been diagnosed with COPD — after all, they figure, the damage is already done. This is true, but you can choose to stop causing *more* damage by kicking the tobacco habit. The longer you smoke, the worse your lungs get, and the harder it is to breathe comfortably.

Eating better

You probably know, at least in a general way, that your diet can have a profound impact on your overall health. But what you eat also can affect how your lungs work and how well the rest of your body deals with the effects of your COPD.

For patients who are overweight, losing weight through diet and exercise can make the process of breathing easier. For patients who are underweight, a diet plan that contains the right amounts of proteins and fats can help preserve muscle strength.

A healthy diet also boosts your immune system — an important consideration, because COPD makes you more susceptible to colds, flu, and other respiratory infections.

Exercising

Loss of muscle strength is a big concern when you have COPD, and exercise is the only reliable way to keep your muscles strong. Exercise can't improve your overall lung function, but it can help you get the most out of whatever lung function you do have. It's also a known antidepressant: Exercising boosts your confidence and sense of self-worth and releases feel-good hormones that make you feel better about life in general.

Prescribing medicines to treat symptoms

Your doctor has an arsenal of medications to treat your COPD symptoms, but it's important to understand that none of them will make your COPD go away. Instead, drug treatments are used to keep symptoms under control and to treat sudden attacks. Chapter 8 covers drug treatment options in detail.

If your COPD is mild or moderate and you don't have a lot of sudden attacks, your doctor may prescribe only a fast-acting bronchodilator to ease your symptoms when you do have a sudden attack. Bronchodilators are medicines that help keep the airways open so air can move through them more easily, and fast-acting ones are commonly called *rescue inhalers* because they're used when you're having a sudden attack.

There are also long-acting bronchodilators that are taken once or twice a day as a maintenance medication to keep the airways open. Not all COPD patients need long-acting bronchodilators; much depends on how severe your COPD is and what other health factors may be at work.

Antibiotics and systemic steroids (oral or intravenous) are usually reserved for exacerbations, although inhaled steroids can become part of a maintenance regimen. Remember, too, that antibiotics are ineffective against virus-based illnesses like colds and viral flu, so don't pressure your doctor to give you these drugs when he says they're not appropriate.

Minimizing side effects

Finding the most effective drugs to treat your COPD symptoms may take some experimentation. What your doctor prescribes and how much you take depends on the severity of your COPD and your sensitivity to side effects. Some bronchodilators can make your hands or feet shake, give you heart palpitations, or increase your heart rate. Sometimes these side effects occur because the medicine isn't taken properly, so knowing how to use your inhalers correctly is important. (See Chapter 8 for instructions on how to use various types of inhalers and other delivery devices.)

Other types of bronchodilators can cause dry mouth or dry cough, or even dizziness, nausea, and headaches. (Chapter 8 describes the side effects of various types of COPD medications in more detail.)

Sometimes people experience side effects only when they first start taking a medication, and those effects disappear within a few days. Your doctor may want you to take your meds for at least a week or two to see if the side effects will go away on their own. If they don't, then your doctor may want to pre-scribe a different dose or even a different type of medication.

Side effects can be much more severe if you don't follow the instructions on your meds. Ask your doctor or pharmacist to explain how you're supposed to take each medication, and don't be afraid to ask questions if you don't understand the instructions you're given.

Preventing and Treating Complications

The most common complications for COPD patients are exacerbations, which are often caused by respiratory infections. Just having COPD makes you more susceptible to whatever contagious illnesses may be making the rounds, and you're especially vulnerable to colds, the flu, and pneumonia. Your doctor probably will recommend you get a flu shot every year and a pneumonia vaccine every five years.

If you're allergic to eggs, you may not be able to have a flu shot. Make sure your doctor knows about any allergies you have, and ask what options there are if getting a flu shot isn't recommended.

Wash your hands often and keep a hand sanitizer nearby for those times when you can't wash your hands, especially during cold and flu season. Most hand sanitizers for consumers, available at your local drugstore or major retailer, contain alcohol, so they evaporate as you rub them into your hands.

COPD's cohorts

Although you and your doctor can take steps to prevent some complications, there are others that you'll have to figure out how to treat. COPD rarely, if ever, is the only health concern; usually it's accompanied by one or more other serious health problems. That's why the way your doctor decides to treat *your* COPD and overall health may differ significantly from the way she treats another COPD patient.

Heart disease

COPD's most common companions are heart disease and circulatory problems like high blood pressure. Heart failure is the most common cause of death for COPD patients. In fact, these two health issues are so closely related that just being diagnosed with COPD automatically raises your risk for heart disease by two or three times.

Many COPD patients suffer from a condition called *cor pulmonale,* or failure of the right side of the heart. The right side of your heart pumps oxygen-poor blood from your body to the lungs to pick up oxygen and then to the left side of your heart, which pumps the new load of oxygen in your blood out to the rest of your body. COPD can constrict or even destroy blood vessels, and that increases the pressure against which the right side of your heart has to work. The extra workload eventually damages the heart muscle on the right side, and it becomes less efficient at pumping blood. This relationship between your COPD and your heart health creates a vicious, downward spiral.

Exercise can help both your COPD symptoms and your heart, which is why it's such a critical part of your overall COPD management plan. A consistent exercise regimen can help lower your blood pressure, strengthen your heart, and maintain your lung function.

Weight control and malnutrition

Being either overweight or underweight is of concern when you have COPD. Being overweight increases your risk for diabetes, high blood pressure, and other weight-related problems, all of which can complicate treatment for your COPD symptoms. Being underweight can further weaken your immune system, making you more susceptible to infection, and can put you at risk for osteoporosis and muscle weakness, which makes trips and falls a big concern.

About a third of COPD patients suffer from malnutrition, which depresses your immune system and contributes to muscle weakness and general fatigue. Chapter 11 discusses ways to make sure you're getting enough of the right kinds of foods and how the appropriate diet can affect your lungs and overall health.

Lung cancer

Chronic bronchitis and emphysema are risk factors for lung cancer among smokers; smokers who don't have chronic bronchitis or emphysema have a lower risk of developing lung cancer. This is another reason you should quit smoking as soon as possible. Having COPD is tough enough. You don't want to add lung cancer to your list of ailments.

Acid reflux

Acid reflux (commonly called heartburn) increases your risk of having sudden attacks of severe COPD symptoms. The link between gastrointestinal health and COPD isn't known, but one study showed that, if you suffer from acid reflux at least once a week, you're twice as likely to have sudden COPD attacks. Acid reflux may cause exacerbations through a process called *microaspiration,* in which tiny amounts of your stomach contents travel up your esophagus and enter your lungs, where they cause irritation.

Sudden onset of severe symptoms

Ideally, you and your doctor both would like to prevent episodes called *acute exacerbations,* or sudden attacks of severe symptoms. The fewer of these attacks you have, the better your general health will be. Frequent attacks also are associated with faster progression of COPD itself.

There are things you can do to protect yourself against sudden attacks: Stay indoors on windy, dusty, or high-pollution days; avoid extremely hot or cold weather; don't let people smoke or use heavy perfumes or scented sprays around you; keep away from chemicals and household products that can emit noxious fumes; take extra precautions to protect yourself during cold and flu season. (Chapter 18 provides a list of common triggers for sudden attacks.)

But, even if you do all these things, you still may succumb to a sudden attack. These can be frightening and even life-threatening if not treated immediately and appropriately. Sometimes using your rescue inhaler will stop the attack. Other times, you may need to be treated with antibiotics or steroids or both for an infection; you may even need to hospitalized. (Chapter 16 has information about self-treatment for sudden attacks and guidelines for when you should call for help.)

 Sudden attacks tend to occur more frequently and often increase in severity as you get older and as your COPD progresses. Go over your action plan for sudden attacks with your doctor at regular intervals to make sure you know what steps you should take.

Optimizing Lung Function

No treatment or activity will restore your lung function to the way it was when you were in your 20s — regardless of whether you have COPD or any other lung disease, because lung function decreases naturally as you age. But you can take steps to maximize the lung function you have now, and that will be a primary goal of the treatment program you and your doctor work out.

Increasing your tolerance for physical exercise

Maximizing lung function means exercising regularly. (Chapter 12 covers exercising with COPD in detail.) The key word here is *regularly*. Occasional exercise won't help you meet your goals of being able to live independently and participate in activities you enjoy. When you start an exercise regimen, you have to stick with it: Your motto here is "Use it or lose it."

Even if you start out in a structured exercise program, you have to keep up the exercise after the structured program ends, or you'll lose all the benefits you gained, both physical and mental. A study of COPD patients in an exercise program showed that all improved their physical and mental functions during the program. A year later, those who had kept up with their exercise program still showed the same level of improvement as they had immediately after the structured program, but those who had stopped exercising regularly had significantly lower scores on all physical and mental assessment tests.

Breathing harder during exercise is normal. It doesn't mean you're causing more damage to your lungs — it just means that the work of breathing has increased.

COPD can impair your thinking abilities, and exercise can improve those same abilities. Prescriptions and other portions of your COPD treatment regimen can involve complicated instructions, so the better your mind works, the better you'll be able to do what the doctor orders — and the better you'll be able to enjoy activities like reading, solving crossword puzzles, and so on.

Trying breathing exercises

One of the reasons COPD can be so frightening is that you don't feel like you can control your breathing. This can make you feel anxious or even panicky, which automatically makes you take shallow, rapid breaths, which makes you feel even more anxious or panicky. Controlled breathing exercises can help you take deeper breaths, calming your anxieties and reducing the sensation of being unable to catch your breath.

Interestingly, many COPD patients figure out breathing techniques on their own. Although no one knows why, people who have chronic bronchitis tend to do diaphragmatic breathing automatically, while people who have emphysema tend to do more pursed-lip breathing. But, since most COPD patients have components of both chronic bronchitis and emphysema, both breathing techniques may be used.

Diaphragmatic breathing

Your diaphragm helps draw air deep into your lungs when it expands and helps force air out of your lungs when it contracts. Many people don't use their diaphragm consciously because they don't need to; in normal breathing, a person may not even be aware of the movement of the diaphragm. But when you have COPD, you have a hard time getting air out of the bottom of your lungs, and learning how to do diaphragmatic breathing can help.

You can do this form of breathing lying down or sitting up. It may be easier for you to do it sitting up, because lying down, especially after eating, can put more pressure on your lungs and make breathing more difficult by removing the assistance of gravity. If you're more comfortable, use pillows to prop yourself up in your chair.

Here are the steps in diaphragmatic breathing (see Figure 7-1):

1. **Sit in a comfortable position and relax the muscles in your shoulders and neck.**

2. **Place one hand on your stomach and the other hand on your chest.**

3. **Breathe in through your nose for a count of three.**

   You should be able to feel your abdomen expand, but your chest should stay still.

4. **Exhale for a count of six, contracting the muscles in your abdomen to help force the air out of your lungs.**

   Again, your chest should stay still.

If you find this technique helps you feel more relaxed and less breathless, try to build it into your daily routine. Two or three times a day, for twenty minutes at a time, is the usual recommended schedule.

Breathing bending forward

Some people find it's most comfortable for them to take deep breaths while standing and bending forward slightly. This position — standing and bending slightly at the waist — may help the diaphragm move more easily; bending forward when you're sitting actually may constrict your diaphragm's movement. You can try doing pursed-lip breathing while you're bending forward, too.

If you have trouble with balance or equilibrium, make sure you have something to lean on when you try bending forward to breathe. Bracing yourself against your kitchen table or a countertop or even the back of a chair can provide enough support to let you concentrate on breathing instead of worrying about falling.

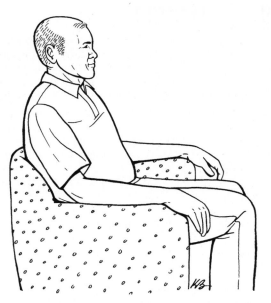

1. Sit in a comfortable position and relax the muscles in your shoulders and neck.

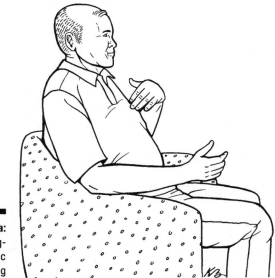

Figure 7-1a:
Diaphrag-
matic
breathing
can help
you relax.

2. Place one hand on your stomach and the other hand on your chest.

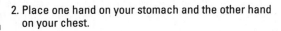

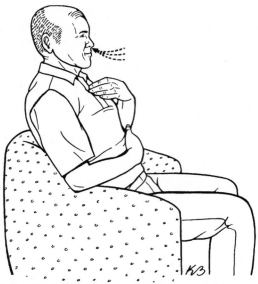

3. Breathe in through your nose for a count of three. You should be able to feel your abdomen expand, but your chest should stay still.

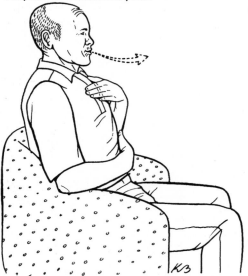

Figure 7-1b:
Diaphrag-
matic
breathing
can help
you relax.

4. Exhale for a count of six, contracting the muscles in your abdomen to help force the air out of your lungs. Again, your chest should stay still.

Pursed-lip breathing

Some people find that pursed-lip breathing is better at relieving shortness of breath and helping them relax. In this technique, you breathe in through your nose and exhale through your mouth, with your lips puckered so that they're nearly closed; imagine that you're blowing on your coffee to cool it down, or that you're about to whistle.

Here are the steps in the pursed-lip technique (see Figure 7-2):

1. **Sit in a comfortable position and relax the muscles in your shoulders and neck.**

2. **Inhale through your nose for a count of three.**

3. **Pucker your lips as if you're going to blow someone a kiss.**

4. **Exhale for a count of six.**

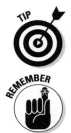

Pursed-lip breathing may be especially beneficial when you're exercising or when you're cooling down after exercising, because it helps you concentrate on getting air out of your lungs so you can inhale more fresh, oxygenated air.

The problem with COPD is that you can take in air just fine, but you can't get it out very easily. The normal ratio of inhalation to exhalation is about one to two; that's why we recommend exhaling for at least twice as long as you inhale, and longer if possible. Taking your time when you exhale helps prevent overinflation of your lungs.

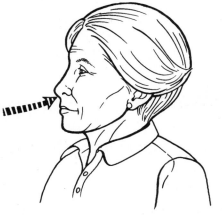 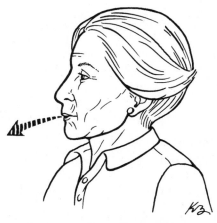

Figure 7-2: Some people with COPD prefer pursed-lip breathing to diaphragmatic breathing.

Sit in a comfortable position and relax the muscles in your shoulders and neck. Inhale through your nose for a count of three.

Pucker your lips as if your going to blow someone a kiss, and exhale for a count of six.

Keeping your airways clear

Mucus — or, more accurately, getting rid of mucus — is often a pesky problem for people with COPD. The disease makes you produce more mucus than people who don't have COPD, and if you allow it to stay in your lungs, it can make breathing even harder. It can also promote infections.

Some of the medications that your doctor prescribes may help loosen mucus in your airways, so you can cough up more of it. Drinking lots of fluids also helps keep mucus thin, so it's easier to cough out. And, believe it or not, regular exercise helps loosen mucus and move it out of the lungs.

Before you start tossing back gallons of water to thin out your mucus, talk to your doctor. Other health conditions may require you to limit your fluid intake, so if you have one of these conditions, you'll need to consider other methods to keep your airways free of mucus.

You can use various coughing techniques to get rid of mucus, and your doctor probably will recommend trying them before considering mechanical devices or medications specifically aimed at clearing mucus.

Postural drainage

The postural drainage technique is common in hospitals and may be part of what your home health aide does for you. *Note:* If you don't have a home health aide, this technique may be less convenient than others.

To do postural drainage, you lie on your stomach on your bed, with your head and arms hanging over the side; your elbows should rest on the floor or on a pillow placed on the floor. Someone — home health aide, spouse, or other family member — claps you on your back to shake mucus loose so you can cough it out. You can adjust your position so the "clapper" can target areas where you feel congested.

Deep coughing

Deep coughing simply means using your stomach muscles, rather than just your throat and chest muscles, when you cough. Using just your throat muscles doesn't really affect the mucus in your lungs; it's more effective for moving mucus in your throat to the esophagus so it can be swallowed. Using your chest muscles results in a hacking cough, which can be very tiring and which doesn't loosen mucus farther down in the lungs.

To do deep coughing, follow these steps:

1. **Sit up or stand up straight.**

2. **Take a deep breath and hold it for a slow count of three.**

3. **Cough using your stomach muscles to force the air out of your lungs.**

Coughing techniques are usually most effective if you use them after you've taken your bronchodilator. That's because bronchodilators, in addition to opening your airways, help loosen mucus, making it easier to cough up.

Huff coughing

Huff coughing is another form of deep coughing; some people find it more effective than deep coughing alone. Some respiratory therapists recommend taking three or four breaths using diaphragmatic or pursed-lip techniques before doing the huff coughing; approaching it this way may help you relax and focus on clearing mucus from your lungs.

Here are the steps in huff coughing (see Figure 7-3):

1. **Sit comfortably and take a few deep breaths using diaphragmatic or pursed-lip techniques (see the "Trying breathing exercises" section, earlier in this chapter).**

2. **Place both hands on your lower chest and take a deep breath.**

3. **Open your mouth and exhale forcefully, using your stomach muscles and making either a *ha, ha, ha* sound or whispering the word *huff* so it sounds like a long sigh.**

   If it helps, press on your lower chest with your hands while "huffing."

4. **Take a few more breaths using the diaphragmatic or pursed-lip techniques.**

5. **Repeat steps 2 through 4 one to four more times.**

Coughing two or three times in rapid succession seems to be most effective at removing mucus. The first cough shakes the mucus loose, and subsequent coughs help move the mucus up your lungs and into your throat so it can be spit out or swallowed.

Inhaling through your mouth after coughing can force the mucus back into your lungs. Be sure to breathe in through your nose after coughing.

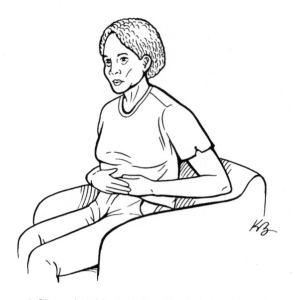

1. Sit comfortably and take a few deep breaths using diaphragmatic or pursed-lip techniques.

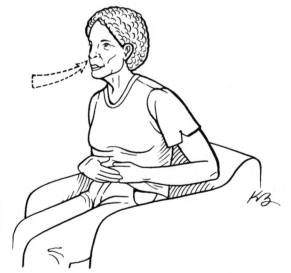

Figure 7-3a:
Huff
coughing
is another
form of deep
coughing.

2. Place both hands on your lower chest and take a deep breath.

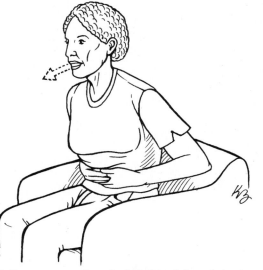

3. Open your mouth and exhale forcefully, using your stomach muscles and making either a *ha, ha, ha* sound or whispering the word *huff* so it sounds like a long sigh.

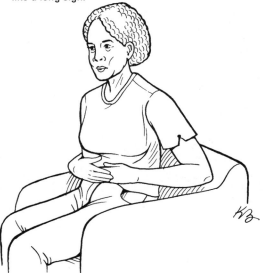

Figure 7-3b: Huff coughing is another form of deep coughing.

4. Take a few more breaths using the diaphragmatic or pursed-lip techniques and repeat one to four times.

Mucus-clearing devices

If coughing techniques don't work well for you, your doctor may recommend a device to help loosen mucus so you can cough it up more easily. Sold under various trade names, these devices produce vibrations in your lungs to shake the mucus free so you can cough it up. These devices include

- **PEP devices:** PEP stands for *positive expiratory pressure.* When you exhale through these handheld devices, they create oscillations in your airways that shake mucus loose. Some PEP devices are used on their own, and some are used with medication delivered through a low-volume nebulizer. Flutter and the Acapella are two brand names for PEP devices.

- **Mechanical devices:** Products like CoughAssist use blowers and valves to apply positive and negative pressure as you breathe through a mask or mouthpiece. These devices also can be used with tracheostomy or endotracheal tubes.

- **Chest-compression devices:** Inflatable vests attach to a generator that delivers bursts of air through a series of hoses. The air bursts create vibrations in your chest, and the vibrations help loosen mucus in your lungs.

Chapter 8

Drug Treatments

Drug treatment for COPD is focused on making breathing easier and preventing — or at least cutting down on the frequency of — acute exacerbations. Medications can help make breathing easier by relaxing your airways and allowing air to flow more freely in and out of your lungs. They also can reduce the severity and frequency of sudden attacks, which can translate into fewer hospital stays for you.

Which drugs are prescribed and their dosage depends on the severity of your COPD, as well as your overall health. The main lines of treatment are *bronchodilators* and *steroids*. Bronchodilators help open the airways, allowing you to breathe in and out more easily. Some bronchodilators work immediately; these fast-acting medicines are used to treat sudden symptoms. Others are slow-acting and are used as a maintenance medication to help keep the smooth muscles around your airways relaxed. Steroids most often are used in short bursts to treat infections, although long-term steroid use is sometimes implemented in late-stage, or severe, COPD.

Antibiotics can treat certain kinds of infection in the lungs (and elsewhere) and help you recover from infection faster. Flu shots and pneumonia vaccines can keep you healthier by protecting you from these common illnesses.

Depending on the severity of your COPD, your doctor may recommend supplemental oxygen. Some patients use their oxygen only when they're exercising or sleeping; others need it on a more continuous basis.

There are lots of ways to take your medicine. Bronchodilators, steroids, and oxygen all can be inhaled; steroids sometimes are taken in pill or syrup form, too. Bronchodilators and steroids both can be administered in powder form through inhalers or in a vapor form through a machine called a *nebulizer*.

In this chapter, we guide you through the maze of drug treatments, showing you what each class of drugs does for you and what side effects you may experience. We also provide step-by-step instructions, with illustrations, on how to properly use the inhalers and other devices that deliver your medicine to your lungs, as well as tips to help you take your medications properly.

Bronchodilators

When the airways are constricted, there can be a buildup of mucus and it's harder to breathe. Bronchodilators relax the bronchial muscles so the airways are wider and the mucus doesn't block air flow. There are several different kinds of bronchodilators, and each type works in its own way to open the airways. This is why some COPD patients take more than one kind of bronchodilator: You can get maximum benefit by combining different types of this medicine.

There are three kinds of bronchodilators:

- ✔ **Beta-agonists** work mainly on the bands of muscle surrounding your smaller airways, telling them to relax and, thus, allowing the airways to open.

- ✔ **Anticholinergics** work on the muscles that surround your larger airways, preventing them from tightening.

- ✔ **Theophylline** medicines also affect the muscles around the airways, and there is evidence that they help your diaphragm work better. Theophylline also has been shown to reduce swelling in the lungs, which can be beneficial for COPD patients. These meds also may help your diaphragm work better.

A word on generic drugs

Generic drugs are often much cheaper than their brand-name counterparts, so it's worth checking with your insurer to see if you can get a break on your co-pay if you use generics. According to the U.S. Food & Drug Administration (FDA), generics contain the same active ingredients and have the same effects as brand-name medications but cost between 30 percent and 80 percent less than the brand-name versions. Generic drug manufacturers have to ensure that their formulations provide the same therapeutic effects as brand-name drugs; their version of the medicine has to enter the bloodstream in the same way and in the same length of time as the brand-name drug. However, because individuals have different responses to medications for all kinds of reasons, generics sometimes have different side effects or interact differently with other medications. Be sure to ask your doctor whether generics are appropriate for you.

Theophylline medications are becoming less common, mainly because newer medications are equally or more effective and often don't produce the side effects that theophylline can.

All three types of bronchodilators come in short- and long-acting forms. Short-acting or fast-acting medications are used to relieve sudden symptoms; they're sometimes called *rescue meds* for that reason. Long-acting bronchodilators are used as maintenance meds to keep the airways open continuously; they can do this for between 12 and 24 hours, which is much more convenient than using a short-acting med every 4 to 6 hours around the clock.

Short-acting bronchodilators

Short-acting bronchodilators relieve symptoms of breathlessness within a matter of minutes, but their effects only last a few hours. The most common way to take a short-acting bronchodilator is through an inhaler, although they are available in pill and injectible forms. Pills and intravenous bronchodilators tend to produce more side effects than inhaled forms. Inhaled short-acting bronchodilators can be administered through an inhaler or in vapor form in a nebulizer.

Short-acting beta-agonists

These medications provide the fastest relief for breathlessness, usually working within three to five minutes. They also can be taken as a preventive measure; if you know you'll be going out into extremely cold air, for example, you may use your short-acting beta-agonist before you go out to prevent yourself from feeling short of breath. Similarly, your doctor may recommend that you use it before you exercise so you don't feel overly short of breath from the exertion.

Short-acting beta-agonists include the brand names Proventil, Buventol, Alupent, Bronkosol, and Xopenex. Generic forms of these preparations are available, too; the most well-known generic versions are albuterol (Proventil) and salbutamol (Buventol).

Typically, your doctor will prescribe taking one or two puffs of your short-acting beta-agonist every four to six hours, as needed. If your symptoms suddenly get worse more often, or you think your medication isn't helping your symptoms, tell your doctor. He may want to change your medication or adjust the dose.

Take your short-acting inhaler wherever you go, the same way you take your wallet and your house keys with you. You never know when you'll need it to treat sudden symptoms.

Short-acting anticholinergics

Short-acting anticholinergics take longer than beta-agonists to work — about 15 minutes, as opposed to 3 to 5 minutes. Because of this lag in relief, they are not often used as rescue meds. However, anticholinergics tend to produce fewer side effects, so your doctor may prefer using this kind of drug to treat sudden symptoms.

Short-acting anticholinergics are available in brand-name and generic versions. Atrovent is available as an inhaler or liquid for a nebulizer; Oxivent is available as an inhaler. The generic equivalents are ipratropium bromide and oxitropium bromide, respectively.

The typical dosage for Atrovent (ipratropium bromide) is two to four puffs, three or four times a day, in inhaler form, or four vials a day with a nebulizer. Oxivent (oxitropium bromide) is usually prescribed for two puffs two to three times a day.

Short-acting theophylline

The effects of short-acting theophylline preparations usually last 6 to 12 hours. Theophylline is usually given in tablet, elixir, or IV form. Brand names include Phyllocontin, Theo-Dur, Theo-24, and Theolair.

Dosage may vary significantly depending on whether you're using a generic version or a brand-name preparation; it's not uncommon for doctors to prescribe higher dosages of generic theophylline products to get the same effectiveness as lower dosages of brand-name drugs. Generally, the upper dosing limit is 800 milligrams a day, but your doctor will need to monitor your dose carefully because of potential side effects (discussed in detail in the "Theophylline side effects" section, later in this chapter).

In general, generics are just as effective as brand-name meds. However, in some instances, such as theophylline (and some antidepressants like Lexapro), the generic equivalent is actually a higher dose than the brand-name version. For instance, a doctor may prescribe 10 mg of Lexapro, but 20 mg of citalopram, which is the generic equivalent of Lexapro. Because health insurance co-pays are based on monthly supplies and not (usually) specific doses, this doesn't affect the difference in price between the generic and the brand-name med: If your co-pay is $15 a month for a generic and $30 a month for the brand name, it's going to be $15/$30 no matter how many milligrams you're taking of either type.

Long-acting bronchodilators

Long-acting bronchodilators last between 12 and 24 hours and are considered maintenance medications; that is, you take them regularly, regardless of whether you have any symptoms, to keep your airways open. When you use your long-acting bronchodilators properly, you may sleep better and find you don't have to use your reliever medications as often.

Long-acting beta-agonists

Beta-agonists that last 12 hours or more are fairly new, so there are only a few versions currently available. Formoterol, sold generically and under the brand names Oxis and Foradil, has both short- and long-acting properties, but is prescribed — and should be used — only as a long-acting bronchodilator. It begins to take effect after about 20 minutes and lasts about 12 hours.

When we talk about generic drugs, we're actually referring to the active ingredient — the ingredient that creates the beneficial health effects — so it's not unusual for one generic to be common to two or more brands. Think of pain relievers: Aspirin, ibuprofen, and acetaminophen are all generics, while Bayer and St. John's, Advil and Motrin, and Tylenol and Exdol are respective brand names for those generics.

Do *not* use formoterol as a rescue med. Because it has long-lasting properties, it should not be taken more than twice a day. Overdoses can lead to severe, even life-threatening, breathing problems.

The other form of long-acting beta-agonist, salmeterol, works only as a maintenance bronchodilator. Like formoterol, it takes about 20 minutes to begin working and lasts about 12 hours. Salmeterol is available generically and under the brand name Serevent.

Depending on the formulation, you take one or two puffs of your long-acting beta-agonist in the morning and again in the evening.

Long-acting anticholinergics

There's only one long-acting anticholinergic medication available so far, and that's tiotropium, sold under the brand name Spiriva. It's administered in a dry-powder inhaler (you can find details on different kinds of inhalers in the "Using Inhalers Properly" section, later in this chapter). Tritropium works in about 20 minutes, but its effects last for 24 hours, so you only have to take it once a day.

Long-acting theophyllines

Some theophylline formulations last up to 24 hours. These are given in capsule or liquid form, either under brand names like Theo-24 and Theochron SR or as generics. As with the short-acting forms, long-acting theophyllines have to be monitored carefully because of the risk for serious side effects (detailed in the "Theophylline side effects" section, later in this chapter).

These drugs are most effective when taken on an empty stomach, but they can be taken with food if they cause nausea or stomach upset. They should be taken at the same time every day to maintain the levels of the drug in your bloodstream.

If you find the theophylline capsules hard to swallow, you can break the capsule open and mix its contents with a little jam or peanut butter. Just remember to swallow the jam or peanut butter without chewing.

Common side effects

Virtually all medications have the potential for unpleasant side effects. Even the ubiquitous aspirin can upset the stomach, and prolonged use of other painkillers like acetaminophen and ibuprofen can cause kidney problems. Bronchodilators are no exception. Each type, whether short- or long-acting, can cause side effects in a substantial number of people.

Beta-agonist side effects

Beta-agonists work on the muscles around your airways, but they also can affect other muscles — specifically the muscles of your heart and around your bones. You may experience *palpitations,* or a fluttering sensation in your chest. Your heart may start beating faster. You may get cramps or experience shaking in your feet, legs, or hands.

When two or more of these side effects occur together, it tends to raise your anxiety level, which in turn can make breathing more difficult. If this happens, don't reach for more of your beta-agonist. If you feel that this is a minor episode of breathing discomfort, practice your controlled breathing exercises (see Chapter 7).

If you experience moderate or severe distress after taking your beta-agonist, call your doctor or 911. The lack of effectiveness of your beta-agonist can indicate a potentially dangerous acute exacerbation.

Sometimes people experience these side effects when they first start taking beta-agonists and don't have them again after the first few days. For most people, the side effects only last a few minutes. If they don't go away, talk to your doctor; you may need a different dose or a different brand.

Side effects may be a sign that you're taking too much of your beta-agonist, or that too much of the medicine got in your mouth instead of inhaled into your lungs. Don't take more of the medicine than directed, and rinse your mouth with water after using your inhaler (and be sure to spit out the water instead of swallowing it).

Unless your doctor gives you other instructions, short-acting beta-agonists should not be taken more than every 4 hours, and long-acting ones shouldn't be taken more than every 12 hours. Sticking to the appropriate schedule will help you minimize side effects.

Anticholinergic side effects

Anticholinergics have fewer side effects than beta-agonists, which is why some doctors prefer them even though they take longer to ease symptoms than beta-agonists. The most common side effects are dry mouth, which can be lessened by drinking water or other fluids after using your medication, and dry cough. If you have glaucoma, anticholinergics can make it worse. Men who have prostate problems may have trouble urinating.

Theophylline side effects

Theophylline medications can produce serious side effects, which is why dosage must be monitored carefully. If you take these kinds of drugs, your doctor should order regular blood tests to make sure your theophylline levels are within safe ranges.

Side effects with this type of medication include nausea, headaches, dizziness, heartburn or stomach pain, and loss of appetite. You also may feel restless or have trembling in your limbs; you may feel nervous or edgy or have trouble sleeping.

If you have an irregular heartbeat, vomiting, or seizures, call for emergency help immediately. Tell emergency responders that you're taking theophylline medicine, the dosage, and when you last took it.

Steroids

The first thing to understand about steroids is that the ones your doctor may describe for your COPD are not the same as the "juice" steroids you're accustomed to hearing about in connection with professional sports. *Anabolic steroids* are the illegal substances used by some athletes to boost performance and build muscle mass. The steroids your doctor uses to treat COPD are similar to *cortisol,* a substance your body manufactures to protect itself under stress. These steroid medications are called *corticosteroids* to denote their relation to cortisol and the *cortex,* or outer covering, of the adrenal gland, which makes cortisol.

Corticosteroids are effective at reducing swelling and mucus production in the lungs. In asthma patients, these medications are used to decrease inflammation in the airways. In COPD, they're usually used to treat acute exacerbations, which often are triggered by an infection. When COPD is in its very severe stages, steroids may be prescribed on a maintenance basis; in addition to their anti-inflammatory properties, corticosteroids appear to help other medications work better. However, in clinical trials, steroids produce the best results in two-week treatment courses.

If you've been on steroids for a long time, don't stop taking them suddenly; your body needs time to adjust to the withdrawal and start producing its own cortisol again. Always consult your doctor before discontinuing any medication.

Long-term use of steroids seems to be most beneficial in people with advanced COPD; there isn't much evidence showing definite benefits for people with mild or moderate COPD. Ask your doctor if steroids should be part of your maintenance meds.

Forms of steroids

Steroids can come in inhalers, pills, syrups, intravenous solutions, and shots. Shots are rarely used in COPD patients. If you need steroids while you're in the hospital, you'll probably start with an intravenous (IV) solution and then move to oral steroids in the form of pills or syrups.

Inhaled steroids are most often ordered when steroids are made part of your maintenance meds. Brand names of inhaled steroids include Flovent, Pulmicort, Qvar, and Advair. (Advair is actually a combination of the steroid Flovent and the long-acting beta-agonist Serevent.) Inhaled steroids also are available in generic form.

Generic oral steroids, including prednisone, are most often prescribed for short periods — two weeks is a typical course of oral steroids — to help treat exacerbations or worsening of daily symptoms.

Inhaled steroids are preferred because they tend to produce fewer side effects than oral steroids. But they don't work quickly. It may take several days or even several weeks to feel better from inhaled steroids.

With oral steroids, the dose may have to be higher to get the hoped-for effect on your lungs. Tablets should be taken in one dose; taking them with a meal can reduce the chances of getting an upset stomach.

Side effects of steroids

Oral steroids tend to produce more side effects than inhaled steroids, either in high doses or in lower doses taken over a longer period. With oral steroids, you may bruise more easily and experience swelling in your ankles or feet. Oral steroids also can promote weight gain (which may be a desirable side effect if you're underweight) and high blood sugar levels (which can be of concern if you're diabetic).

The most common side effect of inhaled steroids is a yeast infection in the mouth or throat called *thrush*. It usually occurs when the medication stays in the mouth instead of getting inhaled into the lungs. You can avoid thrush by rinsing your mouth thoroughly (and spitting out the water) after you take your steroid medication. Using a spacer or chamber with your inhaler (described in detail in the "Using Inhalers Properly" section, later in this chapter) can reduce the incidence of thrush, too.

Steroids also can cause osteoporosis (severe weakening of the bones), cataracts (clouding of the lens of the eye), and high blood pressure.

Withdrawal effects

When you take corticosteroids, your body lowers or shuts down its own production of cortisol. It takes time for your body to adjust to the withdrawal of steroids and ramp up its cortisol production again, which is why you have to slowly wean yourself off steroids.

This weaning process can produce some withdrawal symptoms as your body recognizes and adjusts to lower steroid levels. Muscle and joint pain are common withdrawal effects, as are fatigue, weakness, and depression. Breathing also may become more difficult. It may take several weeks or even months for steroid withdrawal effects to disappear.

If any of your withdrawal symptoms are severe, or if you have breathing difficulty, tell your doctor right away. Also, alert your doctor if you develop a fever or other symptoms of illness when you're tapering off on your steroids or have recently stopped taking them altogether. In these situations, your body may not make enough steroids to help you fight off illness, which can be life-threatening; you may need supplemental steroids until the illness passes.

Combination Drugs

As their name suggests, combination drugs combine two different kinds of medication. Advair is an example of a combination drug: It contains an inhaled steroid (Flovent) and a long-acting beta-agonist (Serevent). Combination drugs are more convenient and can be cheaper, because you pay for only one prescription instead of two. They also promote compliance; that is, patients who take combination drugs tend to take them properly more often than patients who take these drugs separately.

There aren't many combination drugs available for treating COPD. Those that are on the market either combine a short-acting beta-agonist and a short-acting anticholinergic (brand names include Combivent and Duovent), or a long-acting beta-agonist and an inhaled steroid (brand names include Advair and Symbicort).

Side effects of combination drugs depend on what's in them and the dose you're taking. Make sure not to exceed the dosing instructions your doctor gives you; overuse of your meds, whether singly or in combination, can increase the severity of side effects and reduce the medications' effectiveness.

Mucolytic Agents

Mucolytic agents are medicines that help loosen, thin, and clear the mucus from your airways. These drugs are prescribed more often in Europe than in the United States; most American doctors feel there isn't enough clinical evidence to show that they help, and they prefer other treatment options for patients who have trouble coughing up mucus.

The most commonly used mucolytic agent is called *N-acetylcysteine.* It can be taken orally as a pill or liquid, or it can be used in a nebulizer. Nebulized acetylcysteine is a powerful *bronchoconstrictor,* and it doesn't make a lot of sense to use something that tightens your airways when you have COPD, which is another reason your doctor may never even mention it.

If you're prescribed a mycolytic agent, be sure to ask the pharmacist how to take it. Some tablets must be swallowed whole, while others have to be dissolved before you take them. Likewise, some liquid preparations are to be taken orally, and others have to be used in a nebulizer.

Side effects with these kinds of meds depend on which form you're taking. Liquid solutions can cause rashes, nausea, and even breathing spasms. Tablets can cause nausea and diarrhea.

Before you add a mucolytic agent to your med list, talk with your doctor. Other medications may be making it easier to clear mucus out of your lungs, so you may not need this particular drug, too. And you're the only one who can tell whether you need help breaking up and coughing up mucus.

You may notice a change in your sense of taste after using N-acetylcysteine. Drowsiness, runny nose, nausea, and mouth sores are other possible side effects.

If you have any severe side effects — coughing up blood, wheezing or difficulty breathing, or a skin rash or hives, call your doctor immediately.

Using Inhalers Properly

Inhalers — also known as "puffers" or, more technically, *metered dose inhalers* — are the most common way to deliver COPD medications. They consist of metal pressurized canisters that use aerosol to deliver medication directly to your lungs. The canisters are placed in plastic holders that include a mouthpiece.

Unfortunately, inhalers are the most commonly misused medication device. Part of the problem is unclear instructions in the package; part of the problem is the relatively high level of coordination needed to use them correctly. When they're used properly, they deliver medication directly to your lungs (not to the back of your throat), and they're just as effective as nebulizers. In this section, we show you how to use your inhaler properly, both with and without spacers or chambers, as well as how to properly clean your inhaler.

Using an inhaler without a spacer

There are seven steps to properly using an inhaler without a spacer:

1. **Shake the inhaler for 5 to 10 seconds before you remove the cap.**

2. **Holding the inhaler upright — with the metal canister on top and the plastic mouthpiece on the bottom — place your index and middle fingers on top of the canister and your thumb under the mouthpiece.**

3. **Take a deep breath and exhale slowly.**

4. **Place the inhaler 1½ to 2 inches — the width of two or three fingers — away from your open mouth.**

   Figure 8-1 shows the proper positioning.

   Some package inserts have drawings showing the mouthpiece inserted into the mouth. This is wrong. Inhalers deliver more medicine to your lungs when your mouth is 1 to 1½ inches away from the mouthpiece.

5. **Start to inhale deeply and push down on the canister with your index and middle fingers.**

   Breathe in as slowly and deeply as you can; aim for 3 to 5 seconds.

6. **Hold your breath for 10 seconds, or as long as you can if you can't manage a full 10 seconds.**

7. **Exhale through pursed lips, and then breathe normally.**

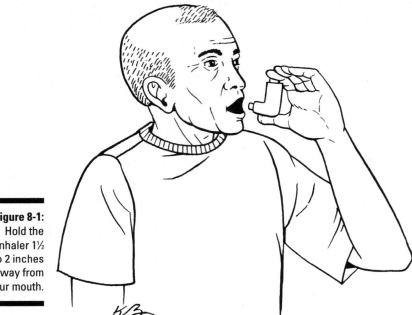

Figure 8-1:
Hold the
inhaler 1½
to 2 inches
away from
your mouth.

If you're supposed to take a second puff, you should wait at least a few minutes between puffs. Ask your doctor how long you should wait between doses.

When you're done, put the cap back on the inhaler. Rinse your mouth with water or mouthwash, and be sure to spit it out (don't swallow it) when you're done rinsing.

Using an inhaler with a spacer

Many people have difficulty coordinating breathing in and pushing down on an inhaler; as a result, they don't get as much medicine into their lungs as they should. Spacers and chambers are devices that make it easier to use your inhaler properly and get the right dose into your lungs.

Spacers and chambers allow you to place the mouthpiece directly in your mouth, which is more comfortable for many people, and breathe in at your own pace. You still get the maximum amount of medicine because it's suspended in the spacer or chamber until you breathe it in.

To use an inhaler with a spacer, close your lips around the spacer's mouthpiece (be sure to remove the cap), press the inhaler button to release one puff of medicine into the spacer, and inhale slowly and deeply for 3 to 5 seconds (see Figure 8-2).

Spacers are sold under several brand names, including Inspirease and Aerochamber. They're all pretty easy to use and reasonably priced. Your pharmacist can help you select one that will be easy for you to use.

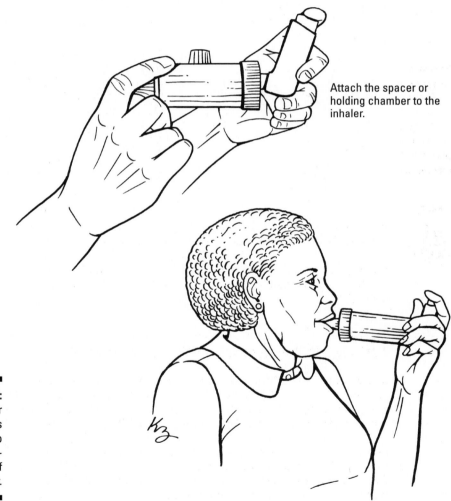

Attach the spacer or holding chamber to the inhaler.

Figure 8-2:
Spacers or chambers attach to the mouthpiece of your inhaler.

Using dry-powder inhalers

Traditional inhalers use aerosol to deliver medicine. Sometimes these inhalers include fluorocarbons, which are harmful to the environment. Dry-powder inhalers eliminate the aerosol component and, thus, the fluorocarbons. (Some aerosol inhalers also have eliminated fluorocarbons.)

Dry-powder inhalers are thick discs with a dose indicator that shows how many doses are left. To use it, follow these steps (see Figure 8-3):

1. **Hold the disc right side up, and slide the thumb grip to the right as far as it will go.**

   Dry-powder inhalers are designed for right-handed users. If you're left-handed, it's probably easier to turn the disc upside down.

2. **Push the lever inside until it clicks.**

   That click indicates that the medicine is ready to dispense.

3. **Seal your lips around the mouthpiece, make sure the disc is level, and inhale as quickly and deeply as you can.**

4. **Remove the disc from your mouth and hold your breath for 10 seconds, or as long as you can.**

Caring for your inhalers

Dry-powder inhalers need to be stored someplace cool and dry because moisture can affect the medicine. Never wash your dry-powder inhaler. If necessary, you can wipe the outside down with a damp cloth and dry it immediately.

Exhaling back into your dry-powder inhaler can push moisture into the medicine chamber. That's why you remove the disc from your mouth and hold your breath; you won't accidentally exhale into the disc that way.

The plastic holders and mouthpieces on traditional inhalers should be rinsed every day in warm water. Let them air-dry overnight on a paper towel or napkin, if possible. When necessary, you can use a mild vinegar-and-water solution to disinfect them; rinse them thoroughly in water afterward so you don't get a mouthful of vinegar taste next time you use them.

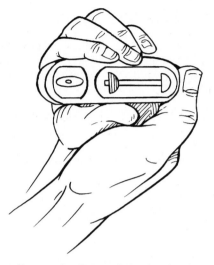

1. To open the disc, push the thumb grip as far to the right as it will go.

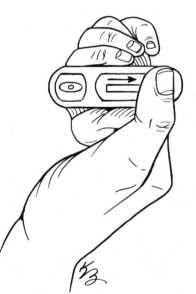

Figure 8-3a:
Using a
dry-powder
inhaler.

2. Slide the lever to the right until you hear a click. The medicine is now released and the disc is ready to use.

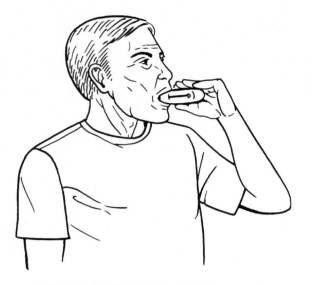

3. Keeping the disc level, seal your lips around the mouthpiece. Inhale as quickly and deeply as you can.

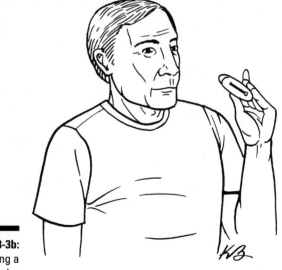

Figure 8-3b:
Using a
dry-powder
inhaler.

4. Remove the disc from your mouth and hold your breath for 10 seconds, or as long as you can.

Using a Nebulizer

A *nebulizer* is a machine, often used at home, that converts liquid medicine into a vapor that can be inhaled directly into the lungs. The machine is attached to a hose and mouthpiece so you breathe in the mist that's created. Several companies make nebulizers, and many health insurance plans cover the cost; check with yours to see if there are any co-pays or restrictions.

Many people find nebulizers easier to use than puffers because you don't have to work so hard to coordinate your breathing and activation of the device. But, when they're used properly, metered-dose inhalers are just as effective as nebulizers in delivering medicine to your lungs.

 Be sure to clean the medicine cup and mouthpiece of your nebulizer after every use to avoid infection. Wash them in warm water and let them air-dry in between uses, or follow the care instructions that come with your machine.

To use your nebulizer, follow these steps:

1. **Put the correct amount of medicine in the medicine cup.**

2. **Place the mouthpiece between your teeth and seal your lips around it, as shown in Figure 8-4.**

   If there's a port, or small opening, on the mouthpiece, put your thumb or finger over it.

3. **Breathe in the medicine.**

   Usually, the recommended technique is to take in several long, slow breaths, resting in between series of breaths. But you can breathe normally if you have trouble doing it the other way.

4. **Tap the medicine cup every now and then to keep the medicine droplets at the bottom of the cup.**

   Your treatment is finished when the machine makes a sputtering noise.

Oxygen Therapy

Supplemental oxygen helps make breathing feel easier. It also can help ensure that your muscles and tissues get enough oxygen, and you may even find that it helps counteract the weakness that so often goes along with advanced COPD. Oxygen is the only treatment that has been proven to prolong life in COPD patients.

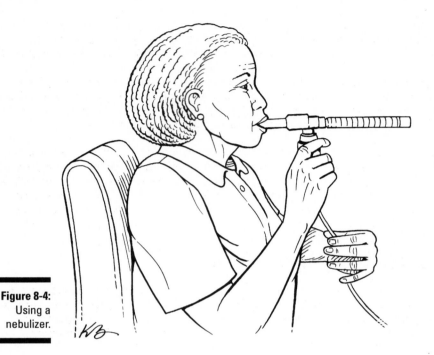

Figure 8-4:
Using a
nebulizer.

Medical oxygen is a drug, just like bronchodilators and other medications used to treat COPD symptoms. It can only be prescribed by a doctor, who may conduct several tests to determine the best flow (prescribed in liters per minute) and the optimum usage of supplemental oxygen.

Oxygen isn't explosive, but it does promote burning. If you're using oxygen therapy at home, enforce a strict no-smoking policy in your house, and keep your oxygen away from highly flammable products like air fresheners, hair-spray, Vaseline, or vapor rubs.

When it's needed

Not everybody with COPD needs to use supplemental oxygen. For some people, it may not be needed at all; this is especially true if your COPD is mild and if you're using diet, exercise, and medications to help control your symptoms. Some people may use oxygen only when they exercise or when they sleep. And some people, especially those with severe COPD, benefit from using oxygen 19 or more hours a day.

People who qualify for home oxygen have to have low levels of oxygen when at rest or after exertion, or indications that low oxygen is causing a strain on the right side of the heart — a condition called *cor pulmonale* (see Chapter 21).

An increase of as little as 1 percent in the amount of oxygen you're able to take in can make a huge difference in how you feel. Using oxygen during certain activities like walking or gardening may allow you to continue doing those things, even if you don't need oxygen at other times.

Sometimes people think if a little is good, more is better. That's not true when it comes to medications, and it's not true of oxygen, either. Too much oxygen can be dangerous. Among other things, it can negatively affect the *hypothalamus,* the region of the brain that controls your heart rate and body temperature. *Never* increase your flow of oxygen without checking with your doctor.

Home oxygen equipment

Supplemental oxygen comes in a variety of systems for home use. Some systems are stationary and can only be used in your home. Others are portable so you can go outside, do errands, and even travel, with a little planning. (Figure 8-5 shows an oxygen concentrator, an oxygen tank, and a liquid oxygen reservoir.)

Oxygen concentrators

Concentrators are stationary machines that separate oxygen from the air and concentrate it for therapeutic use. These machines can be smaller table-top models or larger floor models; some of the larger models are mounted on rollers or casters so they can be moved more easily.

Concentrators are usually appropriate if you use ten or more oxygen tanks in a month. You rent the machine for as long as you need it; check with your insurer to find out if your policy covers the rental fee. Also budget for an increase in your electric bill; concentrators use a significant amount of electricity.

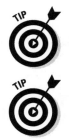

If you're using enough oxygen that a concentrator makes sense for you, have a backup plan for power failures. Keep portable oxygen tanks on hand, or install a generator that can power your concentrator in case of emergencies.

Notify your utility company that you're using an oxygen concentrator. If you run into trouble paying your electric bill, the utility will work with you — and won't shut off your power — if they know you have a medical need for electric service.

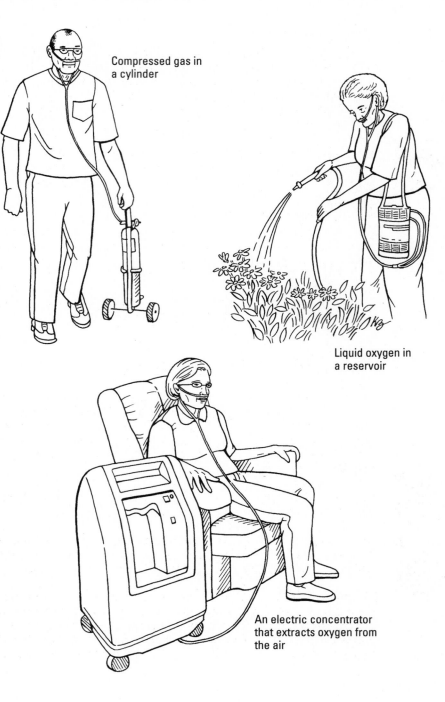

Compressed gas in a cylinder

Liquid oxygen in a reservoir

An electric concentrator that extracts oxygen from the air

Figure 8-5:
An oxygen concentrator, canister, and portable liquid oxygen reservoir.

Oxygen tanks

Oxygen tanks or cylinders are quite commonly used by people who only need oxygen in specific situations, such as for exercising. The larger tanks are not portable; they stand about 5 feet high and weigh as much as an average adult when they're filled. Smaller tanks are used for portability; some models can be pulled along on a wheeled cart and some can even be worn like a backpack.

How long a tank will last depends on its size and your flow rate. As a general rule, you should order replacement tanks when the pressure gauge is at one-quarter full or 500 pounds per square inch (psi, a measurement of pressure).

Liquid oxygen reservoirs

Oxygen becomes a liquid at –295°F (–183°C). As a liquid, oxygen can be stored under little pressure in a Thermos-like container. As it warms up, it converts back into a breathable gas.

Liquid oxygen reservoirs can be large home-based units or small portable ones. The portable units can be filled from your home unit, and they provide enough oxygen so you can leave home for longer periods.

Oxygen delivery systems

There are three main ways to get supplemental oxygen into your body (shown in Figure 8-6). The most common device is a *nasal cannula,* a long, thin hose that connects to your oxygen machine or tank. A foot or two from the end, the hose divides in two, forming a loop with open prongs in the top of the loop that fit into your nostrils; the sides of the loop are tucked over your ears to help keep the cannula in place.

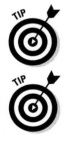

Oxygen therapy can dry out your nose and mouth. Adding a humidifier to your home oxygen system can lessen these effects.

Always adjust the flow rate of your oxygen *before* you put on your cannula. This way, you can check to make sure your equipment is working properly, and you avoid getting a startling blast of oxygen up your nose.

In some instances, oxygen may be delivered through a *tracheostomy tube* (a curved tube, 2 or 3 inches long, that is placed in a surgical opening in the trachea, or windpipe; the tube is connected to a machine that pumps air into and out of the lungs). This procedure is usually used only when there is some injury or illness that prevents normal breathing or swallowing.

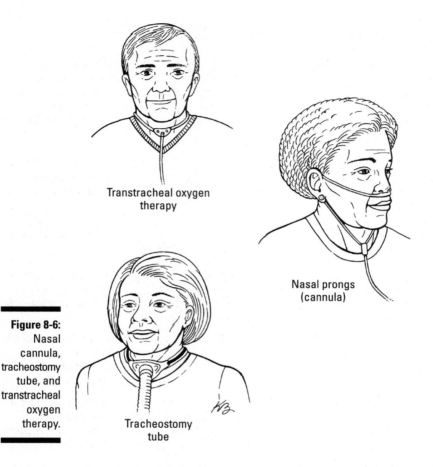

Transtracheal oxygen
therapy

Nasal prongs
(cannula)

Figure 8-6:
Nasal
cannula,
tracheostomy
tube, and
transtracheal
oxygen
therapy.

Tracheostomy
tube

A relatively new technique called *transtracheal oxygen therapy* appears to be more efficient, and more comfortable, than nasal cannulas. A small incision is made at the base of the neck and a small flexible tube, called a *catheter,* is inserted into the *trachea,* or windpipe. Oxygen is delivered through the catheter.

Research indicates that this method allows for true 24-hour delivery of supplemental oxygen and can even decrease the amount of oxygen needed because it's being delivered directly into the airways. Transtracheal oxygen therapy also avoids the irritation of the nose and ears common with the nasal cannula, and it may help ease self-consciousness about oxygen therapy because the catheter isn't as noticeable as a cannula.

Taking Your Meds Properly

A recent report from the National Council on Patient Information and Education indicated that up to half of all people with chronic illnesses either skip doses of their medications or otherwise don't take them properly. That can cause problems when you have COPD: Your symptoms are likely to get worse, you may have severe attacks more frequently, and you may have to make more trips to the hospital.

It also can cost you money. The report showed that not taking your meds properly can add $2,000 a year in doctor visits, and, because most health insurance plans require some kind of co-pay, that means more money out of your pocket.

If you have trouble keeping track of your medications, their doses, and when you're supposed to take them, here are some tips that can help:

- ✔ **Take a list of all your meds to each doctor's visit.** Include any over-the-counter, nutritional, herbal, or vitamin preparations you use — even things like eyedrops and nasal sprays. Write down how often you take each item and how much you take each time you use it.

- ✔ **Ask the nurse or doctor how to take your meds.** Instructions printed on prescription bottles can be hard to read and confusing. Make sure you understand what you're supposed to take and when. Ask if you can or should take any of your medicines on an empty stomach or with food.

- ✔ **Ask if you should take your meds in any particular order.** Especially if you use more than one inhaler, your doctor may want you to take one kind of medicine first. If you have trouble remembering which one comes first, you can use a marker to write 1, 2, and so on, on the plastic holders.

- ✔ **Use one pharmacy to fill all your prescriptions.** When your pharmacist has a record of all the meds you're taking, he can better answer your questions about instructions, interactions, and side effects.

- ✔ **Ask a family member for help.** Your spouse or other relative can help you remember which medicines to take when.

- ✔ **Use pillboxes to remind you not to skip doses.** If you have to take meds several times a day, buy a pillbox that has separate compartments for morning, afternoon, and evening doses.

- ✔ **Use an alarm clock, kitchen timer, or watch with an alarm to remind you to take your meds.** Some COPD meds are meant to be taken at specific times of day. If you have trouble remembering to take your timed doses, use timers or alarms to remind you.

✔ **Don't try to "make up" missed doses.** Doubling doses doesn't help your symptoms and may, in fact, make side effects worse.

✔ **Use a calendar to keep track of when you need refills.** Figure out when your medication will run out, and write a reminder on the calendar to order refills. With most pharmacies and health insurance plans, you can order refills at least a week before you run out.

Chapter 9

Surgery and Alternative Treatments

Surgery is a last resort for treating COPD, reserved only for the most severe cases that don't respond to medication and exercise. The screening process for surgical candidates is intense and involves not just a physical evaluation but often a psychological evaluation as well; surgeons want to make sure their patients are mentally and emotionally able to cope with the unique challenges posed by surgery.

If the primary component of your COPD is chronic bronchitis, you probably won't be considered for surgery. Lung volume reduction surgery and lung transplants are more commonly used to treat severe emphysema; they are rarely used to treat chronic bronchitis. However, because most COPD patients have a combination of the two diseases, deciding who is best suited for surgery can really only be done on a case-by-case basis.

There are some alternative treatments, sometimes called *traditional medicine,* available for COPD patients. Most of the alternative treatments that have been studied are herbal supplements, although there is increasing evidence that properly administered acupuncture can improve feelings of breathlessness and exercise capacity.

In this chapter, we describe the surgical options and the best-studied alternative treatments, and look at the pros and cons of each. Whether any of these options is appropriate for you will depend on your overall health, the severity of your COPD, and several other factors, so, as always, we strongly recommend talking with your doctor before you decide to pursue any of these options.

Surgical Options

Three main surgical procedures are associated with severe COPD: bullectomy, lung volume reduction surgery, and lung transplant. In nearly all cases, COPD patients who are considered for these procedures have advanced emphysema. In fact, *bullectomy* — the surgical removal of giant air sacs — applies predominantly to patients with emphysema, because chronic bronchitis usually doesn't create these giant air sacs. Because surgery to treat chronic bronchitis is so rare, our discussion of these three procedures focuses on patients with emphysema.

Bullectomy

Bullectomy is the term for removing bullae from the lungs. A *bulla* is a giant air sac — *giant* defined medically as more than 1 centimeter (slightly less than half an inch, or about half the size of a dime) — that doesn't contribute to your breathing ability but can make breathing problems worse. *Bullae* (the plural of *bulla*) are believed to form when an obstructed airway allows air into an air sac but doesn't let it back out. Over time, the air sac becomes distended and forms a pocket of "dead" air — that is, air that has very little, if any, oxygen.

Bullae themselves usually don't interfere with breathing, but, if they're large enough, they can compress healthy lung tissue and the muscles in your chest cavity, so the mechanics of breathing are more difficult. Bullae also can impair gas exchange and interfere with blood flow around the lungs.

How it's performed

There are several surgical techniques for bullectomy. Which one is used depends, in part, on how many bullae have to be removed and how large they are and, in part, on the experience and preference of the surgeon.

The least-invasive technique is called *video thorasoscopy.* The surgeon makes several small incisions in the side of the chest (the side with the affected lung, naturally) and uses a tiny camera on flexible tubing to locate the bulla and guide surgical instruments. The bulla is removed through one of the incisions. This is the preferred technique when only one lung has bullae and when there aren't very many bullae to remove.

Another technique, called *muscle-sparing thoracotomy,* requires a larger incision — between 4 and 6 inches long — usually on the side, just underneath the armpit. The bulla is removed through that incision. The technique is called "muscle-sparing" because it puts less stress on the muscles of the chest wall than traditional open-chest surgery.

If there are bullae on both lungs, the preferred technique is something called *median sternotomy,* or what most people think of when they use the term *open heart surgery.* An incision is made along the *sternum,* or breast bone, and the bone itself is "cracked" to give the surgeon access to the heart and lungs.

If there are several bullae and it's hard to define where they end and where healthy lung tissue begins, the surgeon may do something called a *wedge resection.* This involves removing a wedge-shaped section of the affected lung. If an entire lobe of the lung is affected, the surgeon may remove it in a procedure called a *lobectomy.*

Wedge resections only apply to segments smaller than a lobe. Lobectomy is the removal of an entire lobe. Your right lung has three lobes, and your left lung, which is smaller to accommodate the heart, has two.

The benefits

When bullae are removed, the pressure they exert on the lung is removed and the lung is able to expand and contract more freely. The healthy air sacs can do their jobs better, too.

Bullectomy also can result in lower pulmonary blood pressure and less resistance in the airways. With the bullae out of the way, the link between your chest wall and your healthier lung is restored, and your diaphragm can move back up into a more efficient position, which helps make breathing easier.

Most patients who have this procedure are able to exhale more forcefully, so they don't experience shortness of breath as much, and their bodies are better able to carry oxygen to muscles and organs. Bullectomy patients also report a better quality of life, and these effects hold for about three years after the operation.

When it's appropriate

Bullectomy usually is most successful when a large bulla is taking up a significant amount of space in the affected side of your chest cavity — usually 30 percent or more. Your doctor also may want to consider bullectomy if you have pain from a bulla, or if the affected lung suddenly collapses (a condition called *pneumothorax)* when there's no injury to explain it.

If you're coughing up blood, or if you get frequent infections in the bulla, and these conditions don't improve with medication, your doctor also may consider bullectomy.

When it won't help

If you have several smaller bullae, or if there's advanced emphysema in the surrounding lung, bullectomy probably isn't a good option for you. Other health factors, including heart disease, can affect your suitability for bullectomy, too. And, if you have severe breathing difficulties or high levels of carbon dioxide in your blood, the surgery becomes so risky that most doctors won't consider it.

Any surgery carries a certain amount of risk. With bullectomy, possible complications may include the need for a ventilator for some time after surgery, air leaks (common in any lung surgery) that may require a lengthy hospital stay with a chest tube, and development of pneumonia or other respiratory infections.

Lung volume reduction surgery

As in bullectomy, lung volume reduction surgery (LVRS) removes damaged lung tissue and gives the healthier parts of the lungs more room to do their job. Up to 30 percent of the lung is removed, allowing the diaphragm to move closer to its optimal position so it can help more with breathing. LVRS can be used as an alternative to a lung transplant or as a bridge treatment to help patients while they wait for a donor lung.

How it's performed

LVRS can be performed in an open-chest operation, in which the lungs are directly visible to the surgeon, or with a technique similar to video thorasoscopy (described in the "Bullectomy" section, earlier in this chapter). In the latter technique, the surgeon makes several small incisions, about an inch long, and uses tiny cameras and lasers to remove the damaged lung tissue.

Operating on lungs damaged by emphysema is like trying to cut through thin toilet paper. Although surgeons use fabric, dissolving sutures, and even surgical staples to connect the remaining lung tissue, air leaks are inevitable, so a chest tube is inserted to prevent the lung from collapsing. In many cases, the chest tube can be removed about a week after surgery, but some patients heal more slowly and experience prolonged air leaks.

The benefits

In the 1990s, the National Institutes of Health conducted a nationwide study to determine the benefits of treating emphysema with LVRS and other treatments; the study found that the combination of LVRS and medical therapy was more beneficial than medical therapy alone for patients who had emphysema (especially in the upper lobes of the lungs) and low capacity for exercise. Those patients functioned better two years after the surgery.

When it's appropriate

Like bullectomy, LVRS can significantly improve your breathing ability, your tolerance for exertion, and your overall quality of life. But, also like bullectomy, LVRS isn't for everyone.

The NIH study, called the National Emphysema Treatment Trial (NETT), identified which patients are most likely to benefit from LVRS and which are more likely to do worse. Patients best suited for this surgery:

- ✔ Have severe emphysema in the upper lobes of the lungs
- ✔ Have a low tolerance for exertion or exercise
- ✔ Do not respond to medication

Health insurance companies and hospitals often have their own requirements in considering patients for LVRS. Typical requirements include

- ✔ A history of emphysema
- ✔ Quitting smoking at least four months before being evaluated for surgery
- ✔ No previous LVRS
- ✔ No previous heart bypass surgery

Certain heart conditions (besides bypass surgery) may also make LVRS a poor option; your doctor can tell you whether you're a good candidate for this surgery.

When it won't help

Some COPD and emphysema patients won't benefit from LVRS and may, in fact, be harmed by the surgery. LVRS works best when emphysema is located in the upper lobes of the lungs. When it's predominant at the bases, farther down in the lungs, the surgery isn't as effective. For patients who have a high tolerance for exercise and emphysema in the lower parts of the lungs, LVRS has roughly the same effect on function and survival as medical treatment.

And for patients with non-upper-lobe emphysema and a low exercise capacity, LVRS does nothing to improve function and actually has lower survival rates than medical treatment alone. In fact, if your lung function test results are extremely low, this kind of surgery actually increases your risk of dying sooner rather than later.

Lung surgery of any kind isn't a walk in the park, and LVRS is serious business. It's riskier than heart surgery, possibly because patients have impaired lung function to begin with. The U.S. national death rate from LVRS is between 6 percent and 10 percent, one of the highest rates for any surgery.

Lung transplant

Lung transplants replace one or both damaged lungs with healthy lungs from a donor. Although emphysema patients account for almost 40 percent of all lung transplants around the world, this option remains a last resort for treating COPD, in part because it's so difficult to find matching donors and, in part, because COPD patients sometimes aren't the best candidates for transplantation. It's also quite a risky procedure. Between 5 percent and 15 percent of lung transplant patients die within 30 days of the operation. The five-year survival rate for all lung transplants is only about 50 percent, meaning you have the same chance of living for five years after the surgery as you do of dying within five years after the surgery.

When COPD patients do get lung transplants, the goal usually isn't to prolong life but to relieve unbearable shortness of breath. Your odds of surviving with very severe COPD for five years are roughly the same as your odds of living five years after a lung transplant.

Your healthcare team probably won't even consider you for a lung transplant unless your COPD is very severe and you're at a high risk of dying within a few years without the transplant. The best candidates for lung transplants are under age 65 and have given up smoking at least a few months before the evaluation process. You cannot be too much overweight or underweight, and you must be able to walk.

If you become a candidate for lung transplant, you'll be placed on a waiting list. The average wait for donor lungs is between one and two years. You'll undergo an extensive pulmonary rehab program before the surgery. After the surgery, you'll have even more rehab, and you'll have to take drugs called *immunosuppressants* to prevent your body from rejecting the new lung or lungs. Unfortunately, those drugs also will lower your body's ability to fight off infections, so you may be more prone to colds and other illnesses unless you take strict precautions to limit your exposure to germs and viruses.

The wait for donor lungs is so long because the blood and tissue types of the donor must match the recipient's; lung size also is a factor in compatibility. Without a match, the recipient's body will reject the transplant outright. Even when there is a match, though, your body may still reject the new lung.

Alternative Treatments

It may be worth your while to check out some alternative therapies before you and your doctor start looking at surgical options. There are a few out there that have both folklore and scientific studies to back up their claims, and we look at those in this section.

Of course, you must be careful, especially when it comes to herbal medicines; some of these can interfere with your prescribed medications and even skew the results of lab tests — and they may do you more harm than good. Always talk to your doctor *before* you start taking any herbal or over-the-counter preparation.

More and more doctors are open these days to combining mainstream treatments with alternative therapies, as long as the two styles don't interfere with each other. Ask your doctor if she's familiar with alternative therapies for COPD; if not, ask where you can find out more.

Acupuncture

Acupuncture has been practiced in Chinese medicine for more than 5,000 years, but it has only made inroads into mainstream Western medicine in the past couple of decades. Long thought, at least in the U.S. medical community, to be mainly useful for pain management and treatment of addiction, recent studies have shown that acupuncture, properly done, can be an effective therapy for several specific health conditions, including COPD.

Acupuncture is based on the idea that the human body has a series of channels, called *meridians,* that funnel energy. In a healthy body, the channels are all open and energy flow is balanced. Illness and disease occur when one (or more) of these channels is blocked and the flow of energy is disrupted. Acupuncture uses tiny needles inserted in the skin to reopen blocked channels and restore the normal energy flow.

A typical acupuncture treatment lasts for about ten minutes, and the course of treatments usually lasts 8 to 12 weeks. When it's done correctly, acupuncture doesn't hurt, although some patients do experience stinging sensations or slight bleeding at the needle sites. The risk of infection from the needles is fairly low, since the standard of practice calls for using sterile, disposable needles.

Clinical studies have shown that acupuncture can reduce shortness of breath, improve tolerance for exertion, and even improve results in lung function tests for COPD patients. When it's properly administered by a licensed acupuncturist, the technique can lead to significant improvements in quality of life. For some patients, it may even result in enough improvement that medications can be scaled back or (more rarely) withdrawn completely.

Nutritional supplements

There's some evidence that certain nutritional supplements can help ease the symptoms of COPD. However, it's important to take the claims of any supplement with a grain of salt.

Just because something is labeled "herbal" or "natural" doesn't mean it's good for you. Poison ivy is natural, but that doesn't mean it's a good idea to go out and roll around in it.

Here we look at the handful of supplements for which there is some evidence of their effectiveness.

N-acetyl cysteine

Hospitals use N-acetyl cysteine (NAC) to help treat bronchitis because it helps break down mucus. NAC also may help protect lungs because of its antioxidant properties. Clinical studies have shown that three 200-milligram doses per day ease bronchitis symptoms, although it may take up to six months before you feel the effects.

NAC doesn't seem to have any effect on COPD patients who take inhaled steroids.

Creatine monohydrate

Creatine monohydrate is an energy source for muscles. Its usefulness in treating COPD comes from its ability to improve muscle strength and endurance. Interestingly, it doesn't seem to affect your capacity for exercise; that is, if you have a low exercise capacity to begin with, creatine monohydrate may help you feel stronger, but it won't help you exercise any longer or harder.

Magnesium

Magnesium is a key part of normal lung function, and several commonly pre-scribed COPD medications can lead to magnesium deficiency. Oral magne-sium supplements haven't been tested for COPD patients, so we don't know whether magnesium pills are effective. Intravenous magnesium has been tested and seems to be helpful in treating acute asthmatic attacks, but there is much more uncertainty about its effectiveness in treating COPD.

Magnesium deficiency is a little tricky to diagnose because blood levels don't always reflect the amount of magnesium stored in your body's organs and tissues. Symptoms of magnesium deficiency include loss of appetite, muscle cramps or spasms, tingling or numbness, and confusion or disorientation. Ask your doctor about magnesium deficiency if you have these symptoms.

Glutathione

Glutathione is a tiny antioxidant molecule that lives inside every cell in your body. Most people produce enough of this molecule by consuming the foods that create all kinds of antioxidants — fresh fruits and vegetables. But some people, especially those whose immune systems are not functioning at full power, have a deficiency of glutathione. Intravenous glutathione has been used successfully in cancer patients who were undergoing chemotherapy; the efficiency of oral glutathione supplements hasn't been determined.

For COPD patients, the most effective glutathione treatment appears to be in vapor form. The supplement is inhaled with a nebulizer, and it is particularly effective when used to treat acute exacerbations and infections.

Herbal treatments

Traditional medicine identifies several herbs that ease congestion and coughing, but few of them have been subjected to clinical trials. Among those that have, the most impressive is ivy leaf extract, which, in one study, was as effective in treating chronic bronchitis as the drug ambroxol, which dissolves mucus.

Mullein is an expectorant that induces mucus-producing coughs that help clear the airways. It also is believed to soothe mucus membranes in the nose, throat, and lungs. It is commonly used in traditional medicine to treat chest colds and coughs.

Other herbal cough and congestion remedies include lobelia, wild cherry bark, and eucalyptus. Studies on animals have indicated that these preparations can increase mucus discharge, but no human studies have been done.

Part III

In the Next Breath: Managing Your Overall Health

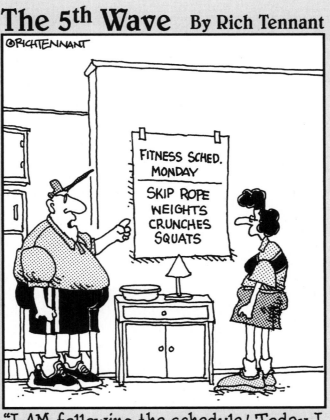

The 5th Wave   By Rich Tennant

FITNESS SCHED.
MONDAY

SKIP ROPE
WEIGHTS
CRUNCHES
SQUATS

"I AM following the schedule! Today I skipped the rope, then I skipped the weights, then I skipped the crunches."

In this part . . .

Physically, COPD affects more than just your lungs. It can lead to weight loss, heart problems, osteoporosis, and a host of other health issues. By the same token, the better your overall health is, the easier it is to manage your COPD symptoms, and the less severe your symptoms will be.

In this part, we address in detail four main health concerns that can affect and be affected by COPD. First, we tackle smoking, not just because it's a strong risk factor for COPD, but because the effects of smoking are so detrimental to your general health. We explain why cigarettes are so addictive, take a detailed look at what smoking does to your lungs, and offer various methods for kicking the tobacco habit in the butt.

Then we cover nutrition, weight management, and exercise — three areas critical to general health and to minimizing the effects of COPD. Proper diet helps maintain your body's immune system and essential functions; we show you how to choose foods that help your body do its job. Because COPD can steal energy from other parts of your body, maintaining the proper weight is important, too. Finally, research shows that exercise can improve your capacity for physical exertion, improve your quality of life, decrease your need for doctor visits and hospitalization, and decrease depression and anxiety. So we show you how to get started, how to set goals that make sense for you, and how to keep track of your progress.

Chapter 10

The First, Best Thing You Can Do: Quit Smoking

As many as nine out of ten COPD cases are attributed to smoking, and the surest way to slow the progress of the disease is to toss the cigarettes. Although you can't reverse the damage to your lungs, quitting smoking means you aren't adding to that damage. And smoking affects more than just your lungs; it also affects your heart and circulatory system, your digestive system, your sleep, and even your cognitive function. The health benefits of quitting kick in as early as 20 minutes after you take that last drag, and they just get better the longer you're smoke-free.

Public policymakers are making it increasingly inconvenient to light up, passing laws that ban smoking in most public places and considering further prohibitions on the practice. Employers are getting into the act, too; some prohibit smoking during work hours, and some even prohibit their employees from smoking at all or risk losing their jobs. And in surveys, a huge majority of smokers — 85 percent — say they would like to quit.

So why do nearly a quarter of American adults still smoke? Part of the reason is that it's so darned hard to quit. It's a physical, mental, emotional, and behavioral battle that many smokers feel they've already lost. For those who started smoking in their teens, the habit is particularly hard to break; a recent study showed that a teenager's reaction to smoking that very first cigarette can set up a lifelong pattern of dependency and addiction that is notoriously difficult to get free of.

In this chapter, we take you through what happens when you smoke — why the nicotine makes you feel good, even while dozens of other chemicals damage your body. Then we look at what happens after you crush out that last cigarette, and we explore various options for kicking the tobacco habit in the butt.

Dying for a Cigarette

Physicians, researchers, and observers of the human condition have known about the harmful effects of tobacco smoke for centuries. As early as the 1700s, some doctors were nagging their patients to leave tobacco alone, and during the Civil War, the *Confederate States Medical & Surgical Journal,* citing the "bronchial disturbances" that smoking was known to cause, opined that "no smoker can ever be said . . . to be well."

Nevertheless, people continue to light up. Smoke-free policies have forced smokers outdoors, perhaps even far away from building entrances; ever-higher excise taxes have been imposed to make smoking economically unpalatable; and anti-smoking campaigns are filled with graphic images of damaged lungs and poignant tales of suffering and grief from the effects of smoking. The scientific evidence of smoking's harmful effects is virtually undisputed. But almost one in four American adults continues to smoke.

Why? Because nicotine makes people feel good, and, like any other addictive drug, it creates a cycle of dependency that makes people crave it more the more they use it.

Smoking significantly decreases your life expectancy. Men who smoke die an average of 13 years earlier than nonsmoking men. For women, the early death rate is even greater: Women smokers die an average of 14½ years earlier than nonsmoking women.

The biomechanics of nicotine addiction

Nicotine is an exceptionally potent poison. It's the active ingredient in certain pesticides, and the amount of nicotine in a single cigarette is enough to make a small child violently (if not fatally) ill. It can be absorbed through the skin (think nicotine patches) or through the mucus membranes in your mouth and nose (think nicotine gum or lozenges, or chewing tobacco), but the most efficient way to get it into your body is by inhaling it.

The nicotine in cigarette smoke gets pulled into the tiny air sacs lining your lungs, where it passes into your bloodstream. Once there, it travels almost immediately to your brain, where it triggers a whole host of neurochemical and hormonal responses:

- ✔ Levels of *adrenalin* (the hormone triggered by danger, deadlines, and other stressors) rise.

- ✔ The higher adrenalin levels prompt the release of glucose into your bloodstream.

- ✔ The neurotransmitter *acetylcholine* (which controls, among other things, your energy level, your heart rate, and the way you breathe) is released in multiple areas of the brain.

- ✔ The high levels of acetylcholine prompt the release of *dopamine* (one of the brain's most powerful "feel good" chemicals) and *endorphins* (the brain's natural painkillers, which, like synthetic painkillers, can induce feelings of euphoria).

All this activity also sparks the release of a neurotransmitter called *glutamate,* which plays a role in learning and memory. When you smoke, glutamate helps your brain connect smoking the cigarette to the good feelings you get from it. It creates a memory loop that tells your brain how to get those good feelings again — a loop that is strengthened every time you light up.

Because of the way it acts on the brain, nicotine is being explored as a possible treatment for certain neurological diseases, including Alzheimer's disease and Tourette's syndrome. The theory is that nicotine may help preserve surviving neurons in Alzheimer's patients and calm the disruptive signals in the brains of Tourette's patients.

Looking at the effects of nicotine on the body

If you're a smoker who can't get going in the morning until you've had that first cigarette, you probably consider nicotine an "upper." If you can't go to bed until you've had one last cigarette, though, you may think of nicotine as a sort of tranquilizer. The truth is, nicotine is both.

The invigorating effect

All the activity that nicotine triggers in your brain energizes your body and makes your reaction times faster. Your heart rate increases; your breathing becomes faster and shallower; and your blood pressure increases. For many smokers, having a cigarette is just as stimulating as drinking a cup of coffee. Indeed, the effects of nicotine and caffeine are similar in that respect.

Nicotine also sharpens your mind, improving your ability to concentrate and, therefore, helping you complete tasks faster and better.

And all this happens within 10 to 15 seconds of taking your first drag of the day.

The sedative effect

Like alcohol, nicotine can act as both a stimulant and a sedative. When you're under stress, annoyed, or otherwise feeling emotionally upset, a quick smoke break can help you feel calmer and more at peace. Part of this effect may actually result from the addiction itself; many smokers go through mini-withdrawals several times a day, and when these mini-withdrawal episodes occur, irritability and tension are likely to increase. When you have a cigarette, you feel calmer because you've resupplied your body with the drug it craves; there are no more withdrawal symptoms — at least for an hour or two.

Understanding why you can't smoke just one

Most smokers can't smoke just one cigarette a day because nicotine doesn't stick around in the body that long. In fact, although an average cigarette has between 8 and 20 milligrams of nicotine, your body will only absorb about 1 milligram when you smoke. The rest of it is broken down and ushered out of your body by your liver, kidneys, and bladder.

For most smokers, the high from nicotine lasts a couple hours at most, and much less for many. That's why smokers often take two or more smoke breaks during the workday, in addition to lunch; it's also why they flock to the exits at airports in between flights and at the theater during intermission. They need to give themselves another dose of nicotine.

The multiple-dosing effect also builds up your tolerance for nicotine, which means, as time passes, you need more of it to get the same level of good feelings from it. That's why people who started out as teenagers sneaking a cigarette or two a week end up being pack-a-day smokers as adults.

Determining whether you're addicted to nicotine

Some people can start and stop smoking any time they want; for some reason, not yet clearly understood, these people don't succumb to the addictive properties of nicotine. Unfortunately, most smokers don't have it that easy. Even when they want to quit, they have to overcome a powerful dependence on nicotine.

If you've made more than one serious attempt to quit smoking but have always gone back to it, that's a strong sign that you're fighting a physical addiction, not just a psychological one. Here are some other indicators:

✔ **You consider whether you'll be able to smoke when you plan activities.** Some people prefer to drive long distances rather than fly because they can't smoke in planes or airports, for example. If you avoid certain places or situations because you won't be able to smoke, it's a sign of addiction.

✔ **You go through serious withdrawal when you don't smoke.** If you get irritable, have problems concentrating, feel overly drowsy, or get headaches when you either try to quit smoking or have to go unusually long periods without smoking, you're probably addicted to nicotine.

✔ **When you've tried to quit, smoking even one cigarette sent you back to your old smoking habits.** The brain's response to nicotine is strong, and it takes a while for the memory loop to close. When just one cigarette causes a full-scale relapse, that's a sign of nicotine addiction.

✔ **You haven't stopped smoking even though it's affecting your health.** Nicotine addiction can be so strong that even smokers who suffer heart attacks, have lung cancer, or are on oxygen therapy just can't quit. If you've continued to smoke even though you have smoking-related health problems, chances are you're physically addicted to nicotine.

Toxic chemicals in cigarette smoke

Nicotine may be a poison, but it isn't the most harmful component of cigarette smoke. Arguably, in fact, the worst thing nicotine does to you is keep you smoking so you can get more nicotine into your system. It's all the other chemicals and particles in cigarette smoke that damage your lungs, constrict your blood vessels, and otherwise wreak havoc on your health.

Nearly 600 additives have been approved for use in making cigarettes. These same additives have been approved for use in food, and they range from the innocuous (apricot extract and bay leaf, for example) to the disconcerting (various forms of ammonia) to the downright disturbing (phosphoric acid — the stuff dentists use to etch the enamel in your teeth when they're putting in a filling).

But it's the burning of cigarettes that creates the most harmful compounds, including at least 40 and as many as 60 compounds that are known to cause cancer. In fact, the Environmental Protection Agency (EPA) lists cigarette smoke itself as a Group A carcinogen, the most potent category of agents known to cause cancer in humans.

Cigarette smoke contains about 4,700 toxic chemicals and compounds, including:

✔ **Carbon monoxide:** The same deadly gas your car exhaust puts out

✔ **Nitrogen oxides:** Also emitted by your car exhaust, among other sources; one of the six principal air pollutants tracked by the EPA

✔ **Hydrogen cyanide:** Used as a genocidal gas during World War II

- ✔ **Vinyl chloride:** Used in making polyvinyl chloride (PVC); banned from aerosol spray cans in 1974

- ✔ **Urethane:** The same stuff they use in varnish, sealants, automobile seats, and other products

Whenever you smoke, you expose the people around you to the same toxins and carcinogens you're inhaling. In fact, secondhand smoke may be even more dangerous because it isn't filtered the way it is when you smoke a cigarette. Secondhand smoke also is created at a lower temperature, which leaves more of the potentially harmful organic compounds intact.

Recognizing Smoke's Effects on Your Body

The real danger in smoking is in the toxic chemicals and fumes that deliver nicotine to your body. Every time you have a cigarette, you subject your body to an assault that affects not just your lungs, but your eyes, your heart, and virtually all your vital organs. When you repeat this assault several times a day for several years, eventually your body loses its ability to defend itself.

Immediate effects of smoking

Your brain may love the feeling it gets when you light up a cigarette, but the rest of your body isn't so crazy about it. In fact, as far as your body is concerned, it's under attack every time you take a drag. Here's a look at what happens to you physically when you smoke.

- ✔ **Gases like ammonia, hydrogen sulphide, and formaldehyde attack your eyes, nose, and throat.** The sensitive membranes in these areas swell in response. Your eyes may get watery while your nose and throat may get dry.

- ✔ **Your lungs start to work harder.** They're compensating for the sudden lack of oxygen in the air you inhale, so your respiratory rate increases. Your airways get inflamed, and your lungs generate more mucus in an attempt to evict the harmful chemicals you've just pulled into your body. You may start to cough; you're almost certainly more likely to succumb to colds, bronchitis, flu, and other respiratory ailments.

- ✔ **Your bloodstream is flooded with carbon monoxide.** Carbon monoxide is a bully that takes over the oxygen receptors on your red blood cells. Oxygen gets shoved aside, and your red blood cells carry the carbon monoxide to the rest of your body.

The perils of secondhand smoke

Secondhand smoke is also known as *sidestream smoke, passive smoking,* or *environmental tobacco smoke.* According to one study, when you inhale sidestream smoke — that is, the smoke that fills the air in between active puffs — you actually may be exposed to more cancer-causing elements than when you actively smoke. This could be because the act of inhaling from a cigarette causes the tobacco to burn more quickly and at a higher temperature, which destroys some harmful compounds.

Those compounds are still present, though, in sidestream smoke.

Secondhand smoke has been shown to cause lung cancer in otherwise healthy, nonsmoking adults. Children who are exposed to secondhand smoke have higher rates of asthma, middle ear infections, and respiratory infections and poorer lung growth and function than children who aren't exposed to it. Secondhand smoke also is associated with sudden infant death syndrome (SIDS).

- ✔ **Your brain and other vital organs become weak.** The lack of oxygen depletes your energy levels. If you're a heavy smoker, your blood can carry up to 15 percent less oxygen than a nonsmoker's blood.

- ✔ **Your heart starts beating faster.** It, too, is forced to work harder to supply oxygenated blood to the rest of your body. In the ten minutes it takes to smoke a cigarette, your heart rate can increase by as much as 30 percent. Your blood pressure goes up, too, increasing your risk of having a heart attack or stroke *while you're smoking*.

- ✔ **Your blood vessels constrict and your skin loses moisture.** You may experience tingling in your fingers and toes because of poor circulation. Your skin may wrinkle and develop a grayish or yellowish tone. Your face may get a leathery look, and you may form deep lines around the mouth, nose, and eyes.

 The things we've just described happen every single time you smoke a cigarette. They may be minor in themselves, but smoking's effects are cumulative. The more cigarettes you smoke per day and the more years you smoke, the more damage your body suffers. The only "safe" cigarette is the one you don't light up.

Long-term effects of smoking

Over time, the minor damage caused each time you smoke can grow into major health issues. According to the Centers for Disease Control (CDC), smoking accounts for nearly one out of every five deaths in the United States every year. Tobacco use — primarily by smoking, but also including "chew" or "dip" — causes more deaths than illegal drugs, alcohol, car accidents, murder, suicide, and HIV *combined*.

Smoking is linked to all four leading causes of death in the United States: heart disease, cancer, stroke, and COPD. It doesn't just hurt your lungs. It hurts your whole body.

Heart disease and stroke

Smokers are two to four times more likely than nonsmokers to develop diseases of the heart and circulatory system, according to the CDC. Smoking also is an established risk factor for *myocardial infarctions,* the medical term for heart attacks.

Smoking can cause heart attacks through several mechanisms. It can lead directly to constriction of blood vessels, including the vessels that supply the heart muscles, which can cause a heart attack. Smoking also leads to damage to the lining of blood vessels, so the vessels are unable to dilate when needed, and that can cause heart damage. Smoking is also a risk factor for developing disease in the aorta — the large artery that distributes blood from the heart to all the organs of your body.

Constriction of blood vessels leads to poorer circulation, which can starve your body of oxygen and lead to the formation of blood clots. Your heart has to work harder to pump blood, and narrowing arteries and veins raise your blood pressure. The walls of your blood vessels can weaken, forming *aneurysms* (balloon-like bulges in the blood vessel that can rupture, causing great pain and even death). Smoking almost doubles your risk of having a stroke.

Cancers

For women, nine out of ten lung cancer cases are attributed to smoking; for men, eight of ten lung cancer cases are caused by smoking. But smoking's cancer-causing effects are not limited to your respiratory system. It also has been linked to cancers of the mouth, larynx (or voice box), esophagus, stomach, pancreas, kidney, bladder, uterus, and cervix. It's also associated with leukemia.

Respiratory disease and other effects

If you're a smoker, you're ten times more likely to develop COPD than a nonsmoker is. Smoking also is associated with a severe condition called *pulmonary fibrosis,* which leads to permanent scarring of the lungs.

Smoking can put both men and women at higher risk for infertility. If you smoke while you're pregnant, you face higher risks for premature delivery, low birth weight, and stillbirth. If you smoke around infants, they are at higher risk for SIDS and for diminished lung growth, asthma, and other respiratory problems as they grow.

Women who smoke after menopause tend to have lower bone density than women who have never smoked. Lower bone density puts you at higher risk for fractures if you fall.

What Happens When You Quit

Every smoker knows he should quit, at least in a vague, it's-bad-for-me sort of way. Part of the problem may be that the rewards of quitting, and even the risks of continuing to smoke, seem impossibly remote from the here and now. Many smokers don't get truly motivated to quit until they've had a heart attack or been diagnosed with a serious illness like COPD. And even then, quitting is no small feat.

The good news is that there are some small but immediate benefits when you quit. And knowing what to expect during withdrawal can help you cope with symptoms when they arise.

How quitting helps your body

The damage done by smoking builds up over time, so it takes your body time to recover from it when you quit. However, there are some benefits your body experiences very quickly after you take that last puff. Your blood pressure goes back to normal in about 20 minutes, for example. The level of carbon monoxide in your blood drops by about half within eight hours, which allows your blood oxygen levels to return to normal.

Two days after your last cigarette, your body will be completely free of nicotine, and your risk of having a heart attack will be lower. You may notice improvements in your senses of smell and taste.

Food is going to taste better the longer you go without smoking, and you may be tempted to eat to compensate for the lack of cigarettes. Talk to your doctor about any concerns either of you may have about your gaining weight.

In three days, you may notice an increase in your energy levels. This is because your airways have relaxed, allowing more oxygen into your lungs and bloodstream.

In two weeks, your blood vessels will open up, improving circulation. It will just continue to get better for the next couple months.

Over the next several months, your lung capacity may improve by as much as 10 percent. Coughing, wheezing, and other breathing problems may gradually wane, depending on how much damage has been done and other health issues.

After the first few months, the health benefits of quitting smoking take longer to show up, because it takes your body time to repair, or at least recover from, the damage that smoking causes. But these benefits are just as critical as the immediate gains:

- After a year of being smoke-free, your risk of having a heart attack is cut in half.
- After five smoke-free years, your risk of having a stroke is the same as a lifelong nonsmoker.
- After ten smoke-free years, your risk of developing lung cancer is the same as a nonsmoker's.
- After 15 years without smoking, your risk of having a heart attack is the same as a nonsmoker's.

The temporary downside: Withdrawal

Quitting smoking means overcoming both your physical addiction to nicotine and your psychological addiction to the act of smoking. Some of your withdrawal symptoms will be physical, but some will be emotional, too, and sometimes it may be hard to tell which ones are more difficult to endure.

Physical withdrawal symptoms

When you smoke, your body changes the way it works to adapt to the effects of the nicotine. When you stop providing your body with nicotine, it takes a while for your body to adapt to the *absence* of the nicotine. It doesn't work the same way it did before you started smoking, and now it can't work the way it did when you were giving it nicotine either. This period between the end of the nicotine supply and your body's adaptation to the lack of nicotine is what causes your withdrawal symptoms.

For most smokers, withdrawal symptoms come out as irritability and nervousness. Physically, your heart rate decreases, so you may feel sluggish or sleepy. This lack of energy may, in turn, make you feel depressed.

You may find yourself eating more. This is partly because, as you recover your senses of taste and smell, food is more appealing to you. Part of it also can be attributed to the jittery feeling many quitting smokers experience; you may eat in an attempt to quiet the craving to smoke.

Nicotine stimulates higher blood sugar levels and decreases insulin production, so many smokers find their appetites diminished. However, although nicotine may increase your metabolism slightly, the health risks are far outweighed by any weight loss you may experience if you smoke.

Psychological withdrawal symptoms

Emotional attachments to smoking are difficult to dissect and almost impossible to explain to those who have never smoked. For many smokers, the habit started at a young age and was a social rite; sneaking a cigarette with friends was both a way to rebel and a way to bond. As adults, those emotional associations with smoking remain. Indeed, as smoking has become more unacceptable in the workplace and public places like restaurants, many smokers may feel a comforting nostalgia in standing outdoors with their fellow smokers, rebelling against the system and forging new acquaintanceships.

So, for many smokers, quitting isn't just about health. It's about no longer socializing with your coworkers over the butt bin outside and no longer making gallows-humor jokes with your fellow smokers outside the restaurant or theater. It's about admitting that your reckless, carefree youth is over. It's about facing the fact that you really aren't invincible, that you don't have all the time in the world left to quit, and that you're the only one who can do this particular task.

Sounds tough, doesn't it? It is. It's so tough that most smokers will delay trying to quit as long as they possibly can. But tough isn't the same as impossible. And knowing what you're up against is, sometimes, half the battle.

Why you should quit, even if you have COPD

Sometimes COPD patients figure there's no real reason for them to quit. The damage to their lungs has been done and can't be undone, so why bother?

It's true that any damage your lungs have suffered so far is very likely irreversible. But continuing to smoke compounds that damage. It gets much worse much faster than it would if you quit smoking.

If you have COPD and don't quit smoking, here's what you can expect:

- **A shorter life:** The average life expectancy after being diagnosed with COPD is five years. It's higher when COPD is caught and appropriately treated early. It's lower when COPD is advanced, when it's improperly treated, and when patients continue to smoke.

✔ **A poorer quality of life:** Smoking adds to the damage your lungs have already suffered, and the more heavily damaged your lungs are, the less you're able to do.

✔ **More complications:** Smokers tend to experience more sudden COPD flare-ups than nonsmokers, and those flare-ups tend to be more severe. Smokers also tend to have more heart and circulatory problems than nonsmokers with COPD.

By contrast, quitting smoking can make it easier for you to stay active because you'll have more tolerance for physical exertion. Your lungs, heart, and circulatory system all will work better after you quit, and you'll feel better knowing you've managed to beat an addiction that gets the best of many smokers.

Trying a Variety of Cessation Techniques

Perhaps because quitting is so inordinately hard, doctors, researchers, and therapists have come up with many different approaches to quitting. The success rates — defined as being smoke-free a year or more after quitting — vary widely, and none of them is surefire. Lots of smokers try at least one or two methods before finding the one that works for them. Here we look at some of the most common and most effective cessation techniques.

Entire books have been written about quitting smoking — what we offer here is really an overview of options. For more information on how to quit smoking, check out *Quitting Smoking For Dummies,* by David Brizer, MD (Wiley).

Cold turkey

Some ex-smokers, and even some experts, think *cold turkey* — just quitting, without nicotine replacements or other stop-smoking aids — is the only effective way to quit. Withdrawal symptoms are intense but usually only last a few days; you can get through most of the unpleasantness of quitting fairly quickly and then concentrate on how much better you feel, which helps you stay motivated to continue being smoke-free.

According to some estimates, almost half of all smokers who try quitting will try the cold-turkey method. About a quarter of those who try quitting cold turkey will succeed — a success rate that's comparable to other cessation methods.

Although some smokers manage to quit by just making the decision to do it and following through, most experts agree that success, even with the cold-turkey method, lies in careful planning, from setting a quit date to changing your routine so you can avoid triggers that make you want to smoke.

If this method appeals to you, here are some tips that can help make it work:

- **Set a quit date.** Make it no more than 30 days out; otherwise, you might lose your resolve or forget. Most experts recommend setting your quit date for a week or two weeks out.

- **Tell relatives and friends about your plans to quit and your quit date.** They'll be more understanding of your withdrawal symptoms and able to provide encouragement. Plus, knowing that you've told everyone about your plans to quit may help you stick with it.

- **Find something to do with your hands.** Keep a straw or pen handy to fiddle with, or take up needlework or another activity that keeps your hands busy.

- **Avoid situations where you're accustomed to smoking.** Ask smoker friends and family members not to light up around you; stay away from places where smoking is permitted.

- **Decide in advance how you'll deal with cravings.** Deep breathing and counting to ten are two popular techniques to get past momentary urges to smoke.

Hypnosis

When it's done properly, hypnosis can be a very effective technique to help you quit smoking; about two-thirds of smokers who try this method are able to quit for a year or more. That's a much higher success rate than any other cessation technique.

The catch is in the words *done properly,* though. Those half-day sessions you occasionally see advertised at a local hotel? They don't fall under the "done properly" heading. That's because, according to research, in order to be effective, hypnosis requires at least four sessions and must be administered according to a specific protocol. And that means you need to consult a licensed psychologist who knows how to use hypnotherapy appropriately.

"Done properly" also means expensive. One session may cost $200 or more, so a full course of four sessions could cost you a cool $800. Of course, that cost is miniscule compared to what you spend on cigarettes and what smoking does to your health, but it may be out of reach for many smokers.

A certified hypnotherapist — sometimes identified by the letters CHT after the name — is not the same as a licensed psychologist trained in hypnotherapy. If you decide to explore hypnosis as an option, you probably won't be as satisfied with the results if you settle for a CHT.

A lower-cost option is a hypnosis audio program. Again, effectiveness depends on whether the program uses the proper protocol. Do your research before you buy; read user reviews online to find out which ones seem to work best.

Antidepressants

Often, people who smoke also suffer from depression, even though they may never have been diagnosed with this common condition. Research indicates that smokers are twice as likely as nonsmokers to have a history of depression over the course of their lives.

In these cases, nicotine may disguise the depression because it stimulates the release of feel-good brain chemicals like dopamine (see "The Biomechanics of Nicotine Addiction," earlier in this chapter). That can make it even harder to quit, because symptoms of depression often return once the nicotine is withdrawn. Smokers who are depressed are less likely to be able to quit, more likely to suffer harsher withdrawal symptoms when they quit, and more likely to start smoking again after having quit for a short time.

There are many kinds of antidepressants, but not all of them are good at helping you quit smoking. Research indicates that two kinds in particular — bupropion (marketed under the names Wellbutrin and Zyban) and nortriptyline (sold under the names Aventyl and Nortilen) — are especially effective in helping people quit smoking, even when patients haven't been specifically diagnosed with depression.

Other antidepressants seem not to be as helpful in the battle to quit smoking. Although researchers don't know exactly why, drugs called selective serotonin reuptake inhibitors (SSRIs), generally don't provide any benefit in terms of easing withdrawal symptoms. Common SSRI trade names include Celexa, Lexapro, Paxil, Prozac, and Zoloft.

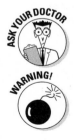

Your doctor can prescribe antidepressants that may help calm your withdrawal symptoms when you quit smoking. Antidepressants can have other side effects, too, so be sure to discuss the pros and cons of these medicines before asking your doctor to write you a prescription.

If you're already taking antidepressants and want to quit smoking, don't try to quit the antidepressant at the same time. You'll essentially be setting yourself up for double the withdrawal symptoms.

Nicotine replacement

Because nicotine, not smoke, is the addictive element in cigarettes, keeping the nicotine in your system is one way to quit smoking while keeping withdrawal symptoms at bay. When nicotine replacement products were first introduced, you had to have a prescription for them, but most of them are now available over the counter.

Nicotine is a poison, and you can overdose on it. That's why most, if not all, nicotine products warn you not to continue smoking while you're using them. If you're using nicotine replacements and still can't quit smoking, talk to your doctor; it may be that you need a higher dose or a different product.

The patch

Your body can absorb nicotine through the skin, so patches are a pretty effective delivery system. Each patch has a set amount of nicotine; you choose which dosage you want based on how much you smoke in a day. You can wear the patch virtually anywhere on your upper body; many people put it on their arm or shoulder, while some prefer to put it on their stomach or side.

Treatment with the patch usually runs eight weeks or more, and the amount of nicotine in each successive week is lowered, so you get weaned off your dependency.

Studies indicate that a combination of nicotine patches and an antidepressant like Zyban work better than patches alone in helping smokers quit. Ask your doctor if this combination makes sense for you.

Nicotine gum

You don't chew nicotine gum the way you chew bubblegum. You bite at it until you feel a tingling sensation; this lets you know nicotine is being released. Then you hold the gum in your cheek until you feel the need for more nicotine, when you bite it again until you feel the tingling sensation.

As with the patch, the gum is offered in various dosages, and you select the dosage based on how much you smoke. Warning labels on the package set a limit of 20 pieces of gum per day, but most smokers use much less. Typically, you use the gum for three months after quitting; maximum recommended usage is six months.

Nicotine lozenges

Like the gum, lozenges deliver nicotine to your bloodstream through your mouth. Lozenges generally come in doses of 2 milligrams and 4 milligrams, with the higher dose recommended for heavy smokers. For the first six weeks, you use a lozenge every couple of hours or so, gradually tapering off after that.

Prescription nicotine replacement products

Your doctor can prescribe other nicotine delivery products, including nasal sprays and inhalers. Nasal sprays get the nicotine to your brain faster than the patch, gum, or lozenges do because the nicotine is absorbed faster through the nasal passages than through the mouth. With inhalers, the nicotine is absorbed through your mouth, the same way it is with gum and lozenges; some smokers prefer this method because the technique is similar to smoking.

There's no evidence that these prescription methods work any better than the over-the-counter products. But many insurance plans won't pay for over-the-counter medications, so, for some people, getting a prescription may make more sense.

Chantix

Chantix, the trade name for varenicline, is relatively new to the smoking-cessation market, so its long-term success rates haven't been determined yet. The twice-a-day tablet has shown a lot of promise so far, though. It costs $100 or more a month, and some insurers won't pay for it because it is so new. However, even if your health insurance won't cover it, the health benefits — not to mention long-term savings — are well worth the expense if Chantix helps you quit.

Chantix works by blocking the nicotine receptors in your brain, so you don't get either the physical or mental boost from smoking. Over time, you lose the desire for nicotine and for smoking, because, without the effects of the nicotine, all you're left with in the act of smoking is the nasty taste and smell.

Chantix does not appear to interact with any other medications, which makes it ideal for people who may also be taking prescriptions for things like high blood pressure, diabetes, or COPD. Potential side effects include headache, nausea, and sleep disruption, usually in the form of peculiar and vivid dreams. Food may taste different, too.

Generally, Chantix is prescribed for three to six months, but your doctor may recommend you take it longer, depending on how you respond to it.

Quitting smoking can heighten symptoms of depression and even thoughts of suicide in some patients, and some medications may make these symptoms worse. Before you take any stop-smoking medication, including Chantix, talk to your doctor about how the med may affect you psychologically.

Behavioral changes

No matter which technique you choose, your odds of success are improved if you incorporate some behavioral changes as well. In fact, some research suggests that your chances of quitting successfully are doubled when you combine one of the options we discuss earlier in this section with behavior modification.

Counseling and support groups can be a great help when you're trying to quit. Your doctor should be able to recommend local support groups. You also can call hot lines at the National Cancer Institute (800-QUIT-NOW, or 800-784-8669) or the American Cancer Society (800-ACS-2345, or 800-227-2345).

Behavior modification is simply a fancy term for changing the way you act when you have the urge to smoke. Most people who try to quit have an easier time if they plan out some strategies in advance for dealing with cravings and for avoiding or responding differently to the circumstances or triggers that prompt them to light up.

Here are some of the most commonly used behavior modification techniques:

- ✔ **Exercise.** Even moderate exercise can help you fight off several common withdrawal symptoms. An added bonus: Exercise is a crucial part of your COPD therapy. A short stroll every day can help ease physical restlessness and help you sleep at night. It also can help reduce feelings of anxiety or irritability.

- ✔ **Practice deep breathing.** Breathing exercises — another critical component of your COPD therapy —can help you feel calmer. Slow, regular breaths signal your body to relax, getting rid of muscle tension. Try to exhale twice as long as you inhale — if you inhale for a count of three, exhale for a count of six.

- ✔ **Stay hydrated.** When you quit smoking, you may experience dryness in your mouth, constipation, and an increased appetite. Drinking plenty of water can help with all these symptoms. Water helps flush your system of nicotine and other toxins. It helps keep your bowels in shape. And it helps you feel satisfied when you're not really hungry but don't know what else to do for your cigarette craving.

While quitting, many smokers find that certain situations trigger an overwhelming urge for a cigarette. Some, for example, feel a strong need to smoke while talking on the telephone; some want a cigarette with their cup of coffee or after meals; some always light up as soon as they get in the car. These triggers are as much unconscious habit as they are true cravings, and most smokers can overcome them by training themselves to think and behave differently. For the telephone trigger, for example, use the telephone in a room where you don't usually smoke, like the bedroom. If coffee seems to make you cry out for a cigarette, try switching to tea for a while, or, if that doesn't appeal to you, try focusing on the coffee itself: Wrap both hands around the cup and concentrate on its warmth and aroma. Develop a new ritual for after meals to replace the smoking ritual. When you get in the car, think about your destination instead of thinking about how you used to smoke.

Write down the times and circumstances when you like to smoke. Then write down alternatives that will help you get past the cravings that these situations will undoubtedly trigger.

Chapter 11

Nutrition and Weight Management

*W*hen you have COPD, you have to pay particular attention to your diet and to your weight. COPD makes your body work harder to distribute oxygen, so you spend more energy just trying to breathe. Without a proper diet, you can't get either the calories or the nutrients your body needs to function.

People with COPD use up to ten times more energy than people with healthy lungs. Unfortunately, COPD often depresses the appetite; when you have COPD, you may not feel like you have any energy to prepare meals, and if you do somehow manage to make yourself a nice lunch or supper, you may not be able to work up the energy it takes to eat it.

Being overweight makes it even more difficult to breathe and can add to your health problems. Extra pounds increase your risk for high blood pressure and diabetes, both of which may complicate efforts to treat your COPD.

Being underweight carries its own health concerns. Loss of muscle mass makes you weaker and less able to get around independently. Your immune system gets weaker, too, making you more susceptible to infections; those infections, in turn, may make your COPD symptoms worse.

In this chapter, we show you why certain foods are better for you than others, and we go into detail about the risks of being overweight and underweight. We show you what a healthy diet looks like and provide tips for crafting a meal plan that works for you. And we look at dietary supplements — the pros and cons of using them and what to look for if you and your doctor decide they're appropriate for you.

Knowing Which Foods Help

An overall healthy diet is an important part of treating your COPD symptoms, but it isn't always enough to follow the federal guidelines on servings of fruits and vegetables, whole grains, dairy products, and protein. Certain foods can help your body ease the effects of COPD, and certain others can make your symptoms worse.

Other health problems that often go along with COPD can complicate your dietary needs, too. Compounds found in red wine and dark chocolate can be good for your circulatory system, for instance. But alcohol can decrease the effectiveness of oral steroids, and simple carbohydrates, like those found in candy, can cause problems with weight and blood sugar levels.

Figuring out the proper diet for you depends on several factors, and you should consult your doctor and your nutritionist for specific dietary recommendations. We can get you started, though, with a look at some foods that can help you breathe a little easier.

Fruits and vegetables

Fresh fruits and vegetables provide a variety of essential vitamins and minerals. They also are high in fiber, which helps you feel full (an important benefit when you're trying to lose weight), aids in digestion, and helps control blood sugar and cholesterol.

Fruits and vegetables are good sources of various *antioxidants*. These nutrients travel throughout your body, seeking out unstable molecules known as *free radicals* and preventing them from causing damage to cells and tissue. Antioxidants include vitamins C and E, carotenoids, and flavonoids.

Vitamin C

Vitamin C is the most common of the antioxidant nutrients that coat the surface of your airways, and research shows that people who take in more vitamin C have less severe declines in their lung function as they age. Eating more foods high in vitamin C may reduce the risk of COPD for those who don't have it, and it may help preserve your lung function if you already have COPD.

Foods rich in vitamin C include citrus fruits (and juices) like oranges and grapefruit. Kiwi and strawberries also are good sources of vitamin C, as are peppers and tomatoes.

Vitamin E

Vitamin E also is critical to lung health. This antioxidant is believed to prevent lung cancer by causing cancerous cells to "commit suicide." It's also known to help ward off respiratory infections and bolster your immune system.

Foods rich in vitamin E include almonds and various seeds like sunflower, whole grains, turnip greens, vegetable oil, and mango.

If you take a vitamin E supplement, look for a mix of *tocopherols* and *tocotrienols*. These are different forms of the vitamin, and your body uses vitamin E most efficiently when both forms are present.

Don't take more than 200 international units (IU) of vitamin E per day. Although proper levels of vitamin E are good for your overall health, some research indicates that ultra-high levels of vitamin E can be harmful. Most people get enough vitamin E in their diets and don't need to use supplements.

Carotenoids

Carotenoids are the pigments found in plants (and some animals). Your body doesn't produce carotenoids itself, but it can use carotenoids from fruits and vegetables to produce vitamin A. Your body needs vitamin A to help its immune system function properly and to keep your retinas and corneas healthy.

Carotenoids are found in leafy green vegetables like lettuce, spinach, kale, Brussels sprouts, collards, and arugula. Broccoli, carrots, sweet potatoes, and winter squash also are good sources, as are apricots, mango, papaya, and cantaloupe.

Flavonoids

Flavonoids are compounds in fruits and vegetables that provide a variety of protective health benefits. Research has shown that flavonoids can boost your immune system, protect against inflammation and allergic reactions, and perhaps even inhibit the formation or growth of tumors.

Apples, berries, onions, and oranges are good sources of flavonoids. Red wine and beer (because of the hops) also provide flavonoids. Dark chocolate — but not milk chocolate — has flavonoids, too.

Consumption of alcohol and sweets may have other health implications, so talk to your doctor before making red wine, beer, or dark chocolate part of your daily menu. Alcohol, in particular, can interfere with your COPD medications.

Omega-3 fatty acids

Omega-3 fatty acids can calm your airways when they're irritated or inflamed. They do this by limiting the production of substances that tell the airways to swell. These fatty acids are found in certain types of fish — particularly wild salmon (farmed salmon has omega-3 fats, too, but in smaller quantities), mackerel, sardines, herring, and anchovies — and shellfish like mussels and clams. Walnuts also are a good source of omega-3 fats, as are kiwis and linseed oil.

Proper levels of omega-3 fatty acids can improve blood flow and overall cardiovascular function. However, if you have congestive heart failure or other heart problems, talk to your doctor before adding omega-3 fats to your diet. Depending on your overall health picture, your doctor may want you to reduce or cut out these kinds of fats completely.

Water

Drinking lots of water helps keep the mucus in your lungs thin, which can reduce coughing spasms and make it easier for you to clear your airways. Most people, including those with COPD, should drink six to eight 8-ounce glasses of water a day.

On the other hand, if you have problems with fluid retention — swelling in the ankles or feet, for example — your doctor may want you to cut back on your water intake.

Water sates us, so we don't feel hungry. That's good if your goal is to lose weight or maintain a healthy weight; drinking plenty of water can help you cut down on snacking. But if your appetite is poor, you may want to cut back a little on your water intake. When you have COPD, maintaining a healthy weight is essential, so you need to do all you can to help yourself feel like eating.

Don't drink beverages during a meal; water and other liquids can fill you up fast so you don't feel like finishing your food. Save that glass of water or cup of tea for after your meal.

Being Aware of Which Foods Can Hurt

Some foods are particularly good for your lungs, but others are best avoided because they may interfere with breathing, contribute to other health problems, or actually harm your lungs. As always, you should consult with your doctor or nutritionist to come up with a dietary regimen that makes sense and is workable for you.

Before you go into that consultation, though, it helps to understand why some foods aren't recommended for COPD patients. Here are some common "problem foods" you should be aware of.

Carbohydrates

Carbs have taken a lot of flak over the past few years, ruthlessly maligned and pushed aside by the advent of the South Beach and Atkins diets. The truth is, your body needs some carbohydrates for energy, and not all carbohydrates are the same.

There is, however, one very compelling reason for COPD sufferers to limit their carb intake: Calorie for calorie, carbs create more carbon dioxide in your bloodstream than proteins and fats do, and COPD makes it harder to rid your body of carbon dioxide. When you're already struggling to take in oxygen and expel carbon dioxide, it makes sense to take precautions against creating even *more* carbon dioxide.

Most physicians and dietitians advise their COPD patients to limit simple carbohydrates — those found in snack foods, for example — and to get most of their calories from protein and healthy fats. So cut out the pretzels and chips, and get your carbs from whole-grain breads or cereals, fruits, and vegetables.

Read the labels on packaged foods to see how many grams of carbohydrates are in each serving. Then limit your carbohydrates to between 15 and 20 grams a day.

Salt and sodium

Too much salt in your diet can make you retain water, which can make it harder to breathe by causing the tissues in your body to swell. Picture a sodden sponge; that's what your muscles are like when you're retaining water.

Salt also is associated with higher blood pressure, which makes sense when you realize that you're retaining water. With all the tissues in your body swollen from water, there's more pressure on the walls of your arteries, which forces your heart to work harder.

Of course, sodium is an essential mineral — your body does need some to function properly — but most people get plenty in their diets and don't need to add more.

If you need to cut back on sodium, try these techniques:

- **Put the salt shaker away.** If it's not on the stove while you're cooking or on the table while you're eating, you're less likely to add salt to your food.
- **Read labels on prepared foods and look for ones that have 300 milligrams (or fewer) per serving.**
- **Use herbs and spices to add flavor, instead of relying on salt.**
- **Cut back on soda, which can contain lots of sodium.**
- **Try using unsalted butter.**

Salt substitutes may seem like a good alternative, but sometimes their ingredients can be just as bad for you as salt itself. See if your doctor or nutritionist can recommend a salt substitute that's right for you.

"Bad" fats

Some fats are essential for proper nutrition, but the so-called "bad" fats — the ones that can clog your arteries and make it easy to put on excess weight — should be limited. This applies whether you have COPD or not, of course, but if you do have COPD, paying attention to the amount of "bad" fats in your diet is even more important.

Why? Because these kinds of fats can trigger inflammation, and inflammation has been implicated in worsening COPD. (COPD patients also often have coronary artery disease, too.) "Bad" fats also are loaded with calories, a big concern if you're trying to lose weight or prevent weight gain.

In the following sections, we cover the two types of "bad" fats: saturated and trans.

Saturated fats

You shouldn't avoid saturated fats altogether. In fact, natural saturated fats — those found in various kinds of meat and oils like coconut and palm kernel oil — are essential to a healthy diet. Saturated fatty acids are the major component of the membranes that surround every cell in your body. There is some evidence that having enough saturated fat in your system prevents stroke; plus, your kidneys need some types of saturated fatty acids to function properly.

But you don't want a diet that's too heavy on saturated fats either. Most people get most of their saturated fats from red meat, poultry skin, and full-fat dairy products like butter, milk, cheese, and yogurt. Talk to your doctor or nutritionist to determine how many servings of these foods you should have per day or per week.

Trans fats

Trans fats are found primarily in processed foods, often in the form of the ubiquitous partially hydrogenated vegetable oil. Stick margarine, many fried foods, and other hydrogenated oils also are rich lodes of trans fats. Tiny amounts of trans fats also are found in some dairy products and meats, but these occurrences aren't usually worth worrying about unless you have some other health issue that sharply restricts your fat intake.

Some research indicates that high concentrations of trans fats in the diet contribute to the incidence of asthma in children. It's believed that these fatty acids affect the lungs because the trans fats are substituted for the natural saturated fats in a special class of cells that cover and protect the surface of the lungs. The trans fats aren't as good as natural saturated fats for this purpose, so the lungs don't work as well.

Hydrogenation is a process used to turn liquid oil into a solid. The heat involved in partial hydrogenation creates trans fats. Full hydrogenation creates saturated fats, mainly in the form of *stearic acid.* Because stearic acid doesn't raise levels of "bad" cholesterol, fully hydrogenated oils are considered less harmful than partially hydrogenated oils.

You don't create trans fats by heating up oil in your own kitchen to fry foods with. However, you can make your homemade fried foods healthier by using butter or coconut oil instead of vegetable oil or shortening.

Nitrites

Nitrites are preservatives used to combat spoilage in cured meats like bacon, salami, hot dogs, cured ham, and meats in prepared meals. Researchers have known for years that nitrites can cause the same kinds of lung deformations in animals that are characteristic of emphysema in humans. In 2007, a study of eating habits and lung disease showed that people who eat a lot of cured meat — defined as at least one serving roughly every other day — had a much higher incidence of lung obstruction than people who never eat cured meats.

Even the researchers who conducted that study said the results weren't definitive, but because cured meats often combine both nitrites and salt, you should limit your consumption if you have COPD.

Potential Problem Foods

There are foods that are good for you that may, nevertheless, cause problems for people who have COPD. Some of these foods may cause bloating or gas, which makes breathing even more difficult; others may promote mucus production; and still others may simply be difficult for you to eat. Here we look at some of the most common potential problem foods and offer tips on how to work around them when planning your meals.

Some COPD sufferers, especially those on oxygen, may have trouble swallowing some kinds of foods. If this is an issue for you, stay away from things like nuts and seeds; granola and certain kinds of crackers also may cause problems for you.

Fruits and vegetables

Full as they are of fiber, fruits and vegetables are notorious for their gas-forming properties. They can distend your stomach and intestines, making it harder to breathe. Baked beans may have the most widespread reputation for causing gas, but they are by no means alone. Common gas-forming and bloating vegetable culprits include onions, radishes, cauliflower, asparagus, broccoli, turnips, cucumbers, cabbage, and sauerkraut. Fruits that can cause bloating and gas include melon and raw apples. Grape juice and carbonated drinks like soda or beer also produce gas and bloating.

On the other hand, you need fruits and vegetables to maintain your overall health and protect your immune system. If you find that certain fruits and vegetables just don't agree with you in any form, stay away from them. Otherwise, try different ways of preparing them. If raw apples cause problems for you, for example, see if baked apple slices are easier for you to digest.

You can also try mixing smaller amounts of gas-forming fruits and vegetables with others that don't cause problems. Instead of just eating a few asparagus spears, chop up one or two and mix them with carrots, for example.

Fried and spicy foods

Greasy, fried foods can make you feel bloated and uncomfortable, so try to limit your consumption of things like fried chicken, French fries, hash, and so on. Heavily spiced foods also can cause stomach problems, which, in turn, makes it harder to breathe.

If you've really got a hankering for something fried and spicy, there are ways you can make these foods more digestible. Instead of frying up hamburger for tacos, for example, try using a mixture of hamburger and ground turkey, and drain the meat well — even blot it with paper towels — before adding your seasonings. This trick doesn't really affect the flavor much, but it does reduce the amount of fat in the final product.

You can use a lighter hand with the spices, too, or substitute milder spices for the really strong ones. Another trick is to pair spicy foods with bland ones: Instead of serving garlic bread with chili, serve plain bread; it makes a nice counterpoint and helps reduce the less-pleasant side effects of the spicy dish.

Dairy products

Milk, cheese, and yogurt are good sources of protein, essential fats, vitamins, and minerals. But some COPD patients have a hard time eating or digesting dairy products. Milk and yogurt may increase mucus production; cheese may be difficult to swallow or may cause indigestion, which interferes with breathing.

Drinking water after drinking milk or eating yogurt can counter the mucus-producing effects of milk. The trick is not to fill up so much on milk or yogurt that you feel you can't possibly drink the water, too. Try splitting your dairy serving in two; drink, say, 4 ounces of milk at a time instead of 8 ounces, or eat only half a container of yogurt at a time. Then you should be able to drink some water afterward.

Caffeine

Caffeine can interfere with some medicines that are commonly prescribed for COPD patients. Too much of it also can make you feel nervous and jittery. Besides coffee and tea, caffeine is present in colas and other sodas like Mountain Dew and in some food, like chocolate.

If your doctor wants you to cut back on caffeine, you have plenty of options. Most coffee brands make decaffeinated versions, and many of them even offer "half-caf" versions with substantially less caffeine. Several sodas come in caffeine-free versions, too.

We aren't aware of any caffeine-free chocolate, so the best advice there is the same as it is for everybody: Enjoy small amounts on occasion, but don't overdo it.

Controlling Your Weight

Being at a healthy weight helps your immune system, which helps protect you from some of the most common problems for COPD sufferers: colds, flu, and other infections. A healthy weight also makes it easier for you to breathe and to move around, so you can do more of what you enjoy in life. Unfortunately, people with COPD typically have one of two weight problems: Either they're overweight, or they don't weigh enough. Each condition has its own effect on COPD, as well as its own risks for your overall health.

Risks of being overweight

Extra pounds put lots of stress on your respiratory system (and your heart), especially if you carry that extra weight around your middle. It can compress your chest wall and crowd your diaphragm, so your lungs can't expand properly and it feels harder to breathe in and out. The extra mass also means your body needs more oxygen but probably has trouble getting it to all your body's tissues.

Being overweight also means you're less likely to exercise, which is vital for COPD treatment. And you're less likely to eat a healthy diet, which means your immune system probably is weaker than it could be.

Finally, although there's some indication that the *obesity paradox* (the phenomenon of obesity, itself a health risk, appearing to provide some health benefit in certain diseases) is at work in COPD, overweight COPD patients are just as likely as healthy-weight or underweight patients to lose muscle mass, not fat, when they do lose weight.

There is good news: Even modest weight loss helps your respiratory system function better, and this applies for those with COPD as well. Lightening the load helps the muscles in your chest and abdomen do their jobs better.

If you need to drop some pounds, the first step is to talk to your doctor or nutritionist about a sensible weight-loss plan. This likely will include an exercise regimen, and it's doubly important that you follow it: Exercise not only makes it easier to lose weight, it also helps preserve your lung function.

Salt makes you retain fluid, so if you need to lose weight, a good place to start is by limiting your salt intake. Your doctor also may prescribe a *diuretic*, sometimes called a "water pill," which helps your body get rid of excess fluid. If you're taking diuretics, you should weigh yourself every day; otherwise, once or twice a week is enough.

Healthy weight loss is slow, around 1½ to 2 pounds a week. If you lose more than 5 pounds in a week, contact your doctor. It could be a sign that something else is wrong.

Everything that causes wheezing is not COPD, or even asthma. When you're overweight, lots of different health issues can make breathing difficult, so before you accept a diagnosis of COPD or asthma from your doctor, insist on a spirometry test.

Risks of being underweight

For many COPD patients, especially those with emphysema, the problem is not weighing enough. It's not uncommon for these patients to lose as much as 20 pounds in a year.

If you're in this situation, gaining weight can pose a couple of problems. The first issue is increasing your calorie intake — essential because you're using so much more energy just to breathe. Your doctor may prescribe a high-protein, high-fat diet or special nutrition shakes like Boost or Ensure to try to raise your daily calories.

But neither the diet nor the supplements will help you gain weight if you don't feel like eating, and that's the second issue for underweight COPD patients. Depression, COPD itself, and some of the medications often prescribed for COPD all can put sharp curbs on your appetite. You may not feel up to preparing a meal, and even if someone else fixes it for you, you may not have the energy to eat.

You can do some things to stimulate your appetite:

- ✔ **Adopt an exercise regimen that's appropriate for you.** Burning energy through exercise can help make you hungry at mealtimes.

- ✔ **Try to eat with someone else.** Most people don't care for eating alone anyway; sharing a meal with a friend or relative can make you feel hungrier.

- ✔ **Make sure every meal includes at least one of your favorite foods.** It will help you look forward to eating, which should spark your appetite.

- ✔ **Perk up your table with cheerful place settings, and put some of your favorite music on in the background while you eat.**

Changing the Way You Eat

Eating is one of the many areas where COPD can force changes you don't necessarily want. We all get into habits, and meals and snacking are no exception, so it can be distressing to feel as though you *have* to adjust your food-related habits. And if you're feeling tired and even just a touch depressed on top of it, you may not even want to think about how to change the way you're accustomed to eating.

It can help to start with the way you think about food. When you have COPD, eating is not just a daily activity. It's part of your therapy for treating your disease. And it's the one part, aside from following your prescribed exercise regimen, that you have full control over.

Eliminating heavy meals

Eating and digesting food require energy, and heavy meals — the traditional meat-and-potatoes fare, for example, or any food that seems to sit in your stomach like a blob — put additional pressure on your diaphragm and chest wall. That combination makes you feel tired and short of breath, which is why many COPD patients feel they don't want to eat at all.

If you want to stick to three meals a day, choose foods that are easy to chew and swallow. This generally means softer foods, like mashed potatoes, bananas, soups, and puddings. When you eat meat or poultry, start with small portions. Three ounces, about as much as will fit in the palm of your hand, is the recommended portion for most people, but you can start with, say, half that and take more if you're still hungry. Take small bites and eat slowly; putting down your fork between bites will help you pace yourself, so you don't get overly tired while eating.

If you're on oxygen, wear your cannula while you eat. Your body is using lots of energy to digest your food, so the oxygen will help keep you from feeling short of breath.

Schedule rest periods before and after meals. Eating and digesting food take a lot of energy, so resting for 15 or 20 minutes before and after a meal (sitting up, of course, because lying down puts pressure on your lungs, especially after eating) can keep you from feeling drained by the exertion.

Adding more, smaller meals

If you can't get enough calories to maintain a healthy weight on a "regular" three-meals-a-day schedule, don't force yourself to stick to that schedule. Instead, "graze" throughout the day, treating yourself to high-calorie mini-meals like whole-milk cheese, crackers and peanut butter, ice cream, pudding made with whole milk, and so on.

Eating smaller portions more frequently throughout the day can help you avoid feeling too tired from eating. Plus, it gives you more opportunities to get the nutrition you need.

An added bonus: You probably won't get as tired preparing your meals, because you won't have to fix a traditional big lunch or dinner.

If you eat more frequently throughout the day, be sure to pace yourself so your last meal doesn't come too close to bedtime. Lying down after eating puts pressure on your lungs and makes it harder to breathe. Plan to eat your last meal or snack at least an hour before you go to bed.

Good-for-you snacking

When you have COPD and abnormal weight loss, snacks that are good for you aren't what you may be accustomed to thinking of as "healthy." No low-fat, no-fat foods for you (unless your doctor tells you otherwise, of course): You need as much calorie and nutrient bang for your snack buck as you can get.

COPD-healthy snacks include ice cream (the good stuff that has lots of butter fat), cookies, pudding and custard (made with whole milk and real eggs), cheese (made from whole milk), popcorn (with butter and parmesan cheese to add calories), breadsticks and cheese sauce, and eggs — however you prefer them, as long as they're real eggs and as long as you eat the yolk, which contains most of the calories and protein in eggs.

What a Healthy Diet Looks Like

We cannot emphasize enough the importance of consulting with your doctor, registered dietitian, or nutritionist to develop dietary guidelines that make sense for you. COPD so often is complicated by other health conditions, like heart disease or diabetes, that it's impossible for us to describe *your* perfect diet.

But COPD can change the definition of a *healthy* diet. Your doctor may want you to cut back on carbohydrates, for example, because your body creates more carbon dioxide digesting a slice of bread than it does digesting an ounce of chicken. On the other hand, you still need protein, various vitamins and minerals, and fiber.

Keeping in mind, then, that your doctor or nutritionist may want you to make specific adjustments, here's what the U.S. Department of Agriculture (USDA) recommends daily for most people:

- **Four to six servings of grains,** such as cereals, bread, rice, potatoes, and pasta. A serving equals ½ cup or 1 ounce.

- **Three to five servings of vegetables.** A serving is ½ cup, cooked or raw.

- **Two to four servings of fruit.** A serving is ½ cup or one medium-size fruit — about the size that will fit in the palm of your hand.

- **Two to three servings of protein,** which includes beef, pork, poultry, fish, peas, some beans, and eggs. (Nuts also are good sources of protein but can be hard to swallow for COPD sufferers.) A serving is between 2 and 3 ounces, about as much as will fit in your palm.

- **Two to three servings of dairy products,** such as milk, cheese, and yogurt. A serving is 1 cup.

The protein you need

Everybody needs protein, but people with lung disease must make doubly sure they get enough protein in their diets. That's because a lack of protein puts you at higher risk for respiratory infections, and you're already at a higher risk for infection when you have COPD. In turn, infections require more energy (in the form of calories) but dampen your appetite. It's frighteningly easy to get stuck in a cycle of having to eat to keep up your strength but not feeling like eating anything because you don't feel well, and not being able to feel better because you're not eating enough to meet your body's energy needs.

Most nutritionists recommend that you eat 1 gram of protein for every kilogram you weigh. To convert your weight from pounds to kilograms, multiply the pounds by 0.45. (A 100-pound person, for example, weighs 45 kilograms, and a 200-pound person weighs 90 kilograms.) When you know your weight in kilograms, you know how many grams of protein you should aim to eat every day. An ounce is equal to about 28.35 grams, so a 3-ounce serving of steak is just over 85 grams (3 ounces × 28.35 = 85.05 grams).

You can add protein to many foods by grinding up nuts and sprinkling the dust over ice cream or pudding, or by adding dry milk, eggs, or powdered eggs to soups and casseroles.

Vital vitamins and minerals

In the proper amounts, vitamins and minerals can bolster your immune system (helping you fight off infection) and protect your lung function. Research has shown, for example, that adding vitamin A — most commonly consumed as beta carotene in fruits and vegetables like apricots and carrots — is particularly beneficial to COPD patients who have a deficiency of that particular vitamin. However, excessive levels of vitamin A can be toxic, so talk with your doctor before taking a vitamin A supplement.

There's no such thing as a bad vitamin or mineral, as long as it's taken in the right dose. For COPD patients, though, there are two areas that bear watching: getting enough vitamin B, and getting enough potassium.

B vitamins

The B vitamins — a class of eight separate nutrients — do lots of things, including helping your body digest and metabolize the fats and carbohydrates you consume. Deficiencies in any of the B vitamins can make you vulnerable to a range of health problems like anemia, high blood pressure, diarrhea, and depression. Proper levels of B vitamins help your immune and nervous systems function well and even help you fight stress and insomnia.

B vitamins are found in a wide variety of foods, from bananas and potatoes to turkey and even molasses. Talk to your doctor about whether you're getting enough of these vitamins in your diet; if not, she may recommend a daily multivitamin or vitamin B supplement.

Potassium

Your body needs potassium for your nervous system, your muscles, and your heart. It helps convey the signals along your nervous system that tell your muscles when to contract and relax; it even helps your muscles do what your nervous system tells them to do. Getting enough potassium also helps keep your blood pressure under control.

If you're on diuretics, or if you have trouble staying hydrated, your potassium levels can fall dangerously low. Symptoms of low potassium levels include muscle cramps or weakness and a tingling sensation in the extremities. If the deficiency is bad enough, you may even experience something called *respiratory paralysis,* in which the muscles involved in breathing are literally unable to expand and contract.

Fortunately, building potassium-rich foods into your diet is easy. Bananas, oranges, orange juice, and fresh pineapple are excellent sources, as are lima beans, split peas, and sweet potatoes. Beef, bacon, sardines, and salmon also are rich in potassium.

Some foods that are high in potassium are also high in salt, like sardines and bacon. If salt is a health concern for you, talk to your doctor about the best food choices for getting enough potassium without upping your salt intake.

Fiber

You need fiber — the indigestible part of fruits, vegetables, legumes, and grains — to help you digest your food. Fiber also helps control your blood sugar and is believed to help control cholesterol, too.

High-fiber foods include fresh fruits and vegetables, dried peas and beans (cooked before eating, of course), rice, and whole-grain cereals and breads. Pasta made from whole grain also provides fiber.

Nutritionists recommend eating between 20 and 35 grams of fiber per day. That's the equivalent of eating a cup of whole-grain cereal at breakfast, two slices of whole-grain bread and an apple at lunch, and a cup of peas or beans at dinner. All of that is in *addition* to the other foods you need to eat to get a healthy diet, and that can be a lot when you have COPD and you don't have much of an appetite. In addition, fiber is filling, so you may find it harder to breathe if you try to get all the recommended fiber in at every meal.

 If you're having trouble fitting enough fiber into your daily diet, talk to your doctor about options. Maybe you don't need as much fiber as is generally recommended, or maybe your doctor would prefer that you take a fiber supplement.

Dietary Supplements

There are literally hundreds of dietary supplements on the market, ranging from garden-variety multivitamins to complex herbal mixtures that you may never have heard of. Lots of them make encouraging, even inspiring, claims about their health benefits. Some of them are beneficial, and some don't do much good but don't hurt. On the other hand, some can be harmful, too. So before you spend your money on these products, there are some things you should consider.

Pros and cons

Although they aren't regulated the same way that over-the-counter and prescription medications are, dietary supplements have the same potential for side effects and negative interactions with your other meds. So it's important to weigh the possible benefits against the possible risks before you embark on a regimen of supplements.

Potential benefits

If you aren't able to get enough vitamins and minerals through your diet, your doctor or nutritionist may want you to take a daily multivitamin to make sure your body has the nutrients it needs to keep you healthy and help you fight off infection.

Supplements can help complement your diet by filling in gaps in your overall nutritional picture. But pills are no substitute for whole foods. For example, there's no compelling evidence that supplements like antioxidant pills are as effective as the foods that contain antioxidants; you shouldn't expect a pill to do for your body what an apple or a cup of carrots can do.

If you're having trouble getting all the vitamins and minerals you need from your diet, your doctor likely will recommend a daily multivitamin and mineral supplement. National brands like Centrum and One-A-Day are generally safe and effective.

Some herbal remedies have been shown to be effective in alleviating certain conditions. For example, glucosamine is often included in treatment programs for certain kinds of arthritis, and research indicates that honey may confer some protective benefits to your respiratory system.

Depending on your diet and other health factors, you may also benefit from specific supplements, like one that provides omega-3 fatty acids. However, because so many supplements can interfere with your prescription medications, don't be surprised if your doctor frowns on your taking any others.

Always talk to your doctor before starting any supplement, and tell your doctor about all supplements and over-the-counter medications you use, even if you don't think they're important.

Potential risks

The U.S. Food and Drug Administration (FDA) does not regulate dietary supplements the same way it regulates prescription and over-the-counter medications. There is no governmental oversight or inspection of the facilities where dietary supplements are manufactured, and there is no standard protocol for making supplements. That means there's no guarantee that these supplements are free from harmful ingredients, or even that one company's vitamin C supplement, for example, is comparable to another company's vitamin C supplement.

Like medications, dietary supplements also can trigger allergies, cause side effects like nausea or the jitters, and interfere with your other medications. They may even make the condition you're trying to treat worse.

In addition, with the exception of multivitamins, the long-term effects of dietary and herbal supplements have not been studied, so we don't know if you run greater health risks when you use supplements for several years.

What to look for

If you and your doctor decide that certain supplements are appropriate for you, there are some things you can do to make sure you're getting what you pay for:

- **Read labels thoroughly.** See what the active ingredients are, how many nutrients are included, and how much of the recommended daily value (listed as a percent under *DV* or sometimes *DRV* on the label) is included in each serving.

- **Avoid high-dosage supplements.** Mega-doses of certain vitamins and minerals aren't good for you. Instead, look for a supplement that provides 100 percent — or close to 100 percent — of the DV for several nutrients. (The exception is calcium because it's too bulky to fit 100 percent DV into one pill or capsule.)

- **Look for *USP* and expiration dates.** The USP designation means the product meets purity, strength, and other standards set by U.S. Pharmacopeia, a testing organization. Vitamins and other supplements also lose strength and effectiveness over time, so steer clear of products that don't have expiration dates and throw out any that have expired.

- **Don't pay for empty promises.** Vitamins and supplements labeled *natural* usually cost more than their synthetic counterparts, but they usually aren't any more effective. Similarly, added herbs, enzymes, or other substances are most effective at adding cost, not any health benefit.

- **Stick with well-known national brands.** According to *Consumer Reports,* which has commissioned independent tests of various supplements, lesser-known brands are more likely to fail tests for purity, more likely to *not* contain one or more ingredients listed on the label, and less likely to pass tests for dissolving properly in the stomach.

Chapter 12

Getting Motivated to Move

. . . .

In This Chapter

▶ Understanding how exercise helps

▶ Relating exercise to other goals

▶ Designing your exercise program

▶ Knowing what's enough and what's too much

. . . .

So you tell your doctor you have trouble breathing, and your doctor runs some tests and says you have COPD, which is why you feel short of breath. Then he looks at you and says, "You really need to exercise."

Say what?

It seems to defy common sense, telling people with breathing problems that they need to purposely engage in activities that will make them breathe even harder. But the truth is that appropriate exercise is a critical component of treating your COPD. It can't cure you, but it can help you make the most of whatever lung function you have left. And that eases your symptoms and improves your quality of life.

An effective exercise regimen combines aerobic activity like walking, cycling, or swimming, and strengthening exercises for the upper and lower body. This combination helps you build endurance and muscle strength, so you can do the activities you like for longer periods and do more of the everyday tasks that often pose difficulties for those with COPD. Exercise also helps boost your immune system, making you more resistant to infection — a continual worry for COPD patients — and helps ease symptoms of depression and anxiety.

In this chapter, we look at how exercise affects your body — not just your lungs, but your heart, your muscles, and your mind. We discuss the importance of setting goals for your activity level. We explore different kinds of exercise, their benefits and their limitations. And we show you how to create an exercise plan that makes sense for you and helps you reach your goals.

How Movement Affects Your Body

Every time you move, you stretch and flex muscles and draw in oxygen to help feed your muscles. The more you move, the more supple and flexible your muscles and other tissues become, so the easier movement gets.

Movement promotes development of additional capillaries — the tiniest blood vessels — around your muscles, providing more access to the oxygen and nutrients in your blood. *Ligaments,* the bands of fibrous tissue that hold your organs in place and connect your bones, get stronger, especially at joints like the shoulders and knees. *Cartilage,* the firm but yielding tissue that cushions your joints, gets thicker, improving its ability to protect your bones from jarring or grinding against each other. *Range of motion* (how far you can lift your arms and legs, move your neck, and so on) improves because your muscles and tissues have greater elasticity. And your bones get stronger, because the cells that make bone material work harder when you work out.

Broadly speaking, there are two kinds of exercise:

- ✔ **Aerobic exercise** helps your body take in oxygen; the word *aerobic* means "with oxygen." Examples include fast walking, running, cycling, swimming, stair-stepping, and so on.

- ✔ **Anaerobic exercise** helps you build muscle strength and overall fitness; the word *anaerobic* means "without oxygen." Anaerobic exercise includes stretching, weight and resistance training, slow walking or dancing, bowling, and similar activities. And, although the effects aren't as dramatic as with aerobic exercise, anaerobic exercise also helps your circulatory and respiratory systems.

Help for your circulatory system

Aerobic exercise helps your circulatory system by strengthening your heart, enlarging your arteries, and promoting the production of red blood cells.

With regular aerobic exercise, the walls of your heart thicken a little, and your heart overall gets a little bigger. The stronger, larger heart can hold more blood and can pump blood out to the rest of the body better. As your conditioning improves, your heart also returns to a resting rate more quickly after exertion.

Your arteries grow a little bit, too, with regular aerobic training. The walls of your arteries also become more elastic. With larger, more flexible arteries, your blood pressure drops, reducing your risk of stroke.

During an aerobic workout, your body requires more oxygen to handle the exertion. That promotes production of more red blood cells to carry the oxygen, and development of more capillaries to deliver the oxygen to hungry muscles and tissues. So you improve your body's transportation and delivery systems for oxygen at the same time.

Help for your respiratory system

Aerobic exercise helps your body make the most of your lung function by strengthening the muscles used in breathing and conditioning you to take in more oxygen and get rid of more carbon dioxide. The longer you participate in regular aerobic exercise, the less frequent your episodes of feeling short of breath will become, and the more endurance you'll build up for different kinds of exertion.

With aerobic training, your diaphragm gets stronger, so it's more efficient in helping you expel air from your lungs. Your *intercostal muscles* (the muscles between your ribs) get stronger, too, so they can stretch more when you inhale; in effect, the improved strength of your intercostals makes your chest cavity larger, enabling you to breathe in more deeply.

As we mention in the preceding section, aerobic exercise promotes development of capillaries, which improves delivery of oxygen to muscles and tissue. This process also happens around the air sacs in your lungs. More capillaries around your air sacs mean more gas-exchange capability; your body can absorb more oxygen into your blood and get more carbon dioxide out of it.

Help for your sense of well-being

One of the biggest issues for COPD patients is depression as a result of forced inactivity, real or perceived. Exercise counters that depression for a number of reasons:

- ✔ It boosts your overall energy level.
- ✔ It builds your strength to take part in other activities.
- ✔ It helps control your appetite.
- ✔ It promotes weight loss.
- ✔ It helps control your blood pressure.
- ✔ It helps improve the quality of your sleep and reduces bouts of insomnia.
- ✔ It improves your posture, balance, and flexibility.
- ✔ Unlike the COPD itself, exercise is something you can control.

Research shows that exercise boosts your self-confidence, reduces stress and anxiety levels, and helps you stabilize your moods. In fact, exercise has been shown to be an effective antidepressant, not just over the long-term, but immediately. And the poorer shape you're in, physically and emotionally, when you start an exercise program, the more effective exercise is in diffusing depression, anxiety, anger, and the effects of stress.

Both men and women reap the psychological benefits of exercise, and older people seem to see more benefits than younger people. That doesn't mean you should wait to start your own exercise program, though; research shows that the longer you engage in regular exercise and the more sessions you engage in, the more it helps you mentally and emotionally.

According to researchers, the most effective antidepressant effect comes from a combination of exercise and some form of psychotherapy or counseling. In other words, while both walking it out and talking it out are good for your health, doing both is better.

For exercise to be effective, you have to stick with it. A study of older COPD patients showed that, after a ten-week exercise program, all participants improved their physical, psychological, and cognitive functions. But patients who stopped exercising after the ten-week program was finished lost their gains in virtually every area the researchers measured.

Always, always, always talk with your doctor before you start any exercise program — not because your doctor will tell you to avoid sitting on the couch all day, but because only your own doctor can assess what kind of exercise makes sense for you. She'll take into account any other health factors that may be in play, as well as your personal goals.

Setting Goals for Your Quality of Life

One of the keys to a successful exercise program is your motivation to do your exercises regularly. It's not enough for your doctor or your family or even us to tell you it's good for you. You have to figure out why *you* want to exercise.

If you're like most people, your reasons for wanting to exercise will have much less to do with the condition of your heart and lungs than with your outlook on your life. And, again if you're like most people, you probably aren't quite sure how to identify the things that really will motivate you to do the things you know you should do anyway.

So, instead of focusing on why exercise is good for you, try focusing on what you would like your perfect day to look like. No, we're not crazy. The best way to zero in on what motivates you is to imagine your life as you would *like* it to be. Then you can figure out what steps you can take to move you toward your goal.

Thinking about what you'd like to do

If you didn't have trouble breathing and you had the energy you used to have, what would you do with your days? Would you get back out in the garden? Go out to lunch with friends? Take in a movie, a play, or a concert now and then? Go for evening walks with your spouse? Go camping? Volunteer at your temple or the Salvation Army?

Thinking in terms of things you'd like to do helps you focus on why you're *really* exercising. Because, let's face it, for most of us, healthier hearts and stronger muscles just aren't the prime motivation. What really matters is how we feel and whether we're able to do what we want to do. If you feel exercise will enable you to do (or keep doing) the things you truly enjoy, you're more likely to stick with your exercise program. And when you stick with it, you're more likely to be able to do, or keep doing, what you like.

Here are some tricks you can use if you're having trouble finding your true motivation:

- ✔ **Remember the past.** It's easy to fall into a bad habit of thinking you'll never be able to do what you used to do. To be honest, that may be true in some cases; if you used to run marathons or play in a softball league or do heavy lifting, you may not be able to return to that level of activity.

  But for most COPD patients, the things they miss doing the most involve social activities. Maybe you used to enjoy playing bridge or poker, but you gave it up because you just don't have the energy for an evening of cards anymore. Maybe you used to have season tickets to the symphony, but you can't remember the last time you felt like going out.

  Think about the things you used to enjoy and decide whether you'd like to do those things again. You may find today's motivation there.

- ✔ **Think about how you feel.** Maybe you long for the days when you used to wake up feeling refreshed and energetic, and your motivation for exercising is recapturing the ability to sleep well. Maybe you really resent not having enough strength to carry a bag of groceries in from the car. Or maybe you just don't want your COPD to define or limit your life now.

  Taking an honest look at how you feel — physically, of course, and how the way you feel physically makes you feel emotionally — can be scary, but it also can be quite empowering. Deciding to exercise gives you some control over your COPD symptoms, and knowing you have some control can be one heck of a motivator.

✓ **Consider what you *don't* want.** Fear is another powerful motivator, and you may be able to use it to your advantage by thinking of the things you want to avoid. For example, if you're not on oxygen now, maybe you want to avoid having to be on it in the future. Maybe you want to stay out of the hospital. Maybe you just don't want your symptoms to get any worse than they already are.

When you've identified the things that motivate you, write them down on a sticky note and post it where you'll see it often — on the refrigerator, for example, or the bathroom mirror. A tangible reminder will do wonders for those times when you can't seem to find your motivation on your own.

Measuring your progress

No matter how motivated you are, chances are good that you won't stick to your exercise plan unless you can see some progress. But, because it'll take time to achieve your long-term goals, you can easily get discouraged and begin thinking your goals are too far out of reach.

Of course, keeping an eye on your main goals is important. But that doesn't mean you should ignore the steps that move you toward those goals. Progress in nearly every endeavor is incremental. Start out with the idea that you'll celebrate small accomplishments on the way to your main objective.

There are several ways you can do this. You can measure your progress by:

✓ **Time:** If you start out walking for 5 minutes a day, try to add 30 seconds or a full minute each week. You could be up to nearly 15 minutes of walking inside 2 months, and that is, indeed, progress.

✓ **Distance:** When you begin exercising, you may feel short of breath after walking just a block or two. After a few weeks, you may be able to walk five or six blocks before feeling like you can't catch your breath. When you can move farther, you know you're making headway.

✓ **Repetitions:** When you first begin strength training in your legs or muscles, you may only be able to do two or three repetitions for each exercise. As with walking, adding a repetition each week gives you a concrete way to measure your progress.

✓ **What else you can do:** Exercise aside, pay attention to little everyday things you can do that weren't so easy for you before you started your exercise program. Maybe it's no big deal now to walk out to the mailbox, for example, or maybe bathing and dressing are easier now. These little things add up quickly to a better quality of life — and recognizing that your quality of life is improving will help you stick with your exercise plan.

Knowing why it matters

Exercise can't reverse the damage to your lungs. But it can do wonders for how you feel physically and emotionally, and it can help protect you from many complications that are so often associated with COPD, such as heart disease and respiratory infections. Regular exercise helps ease COPD symptoms like fatigue and shortness of breath. It helps your muscles use oxygen more efficiently, so your body gets the most out of your lung function. And it helps keep you independent and active longer, less likely to need hospitalization, and less likely to suffer from depression.

Exercise Training

When you have COPD, there are two main areas of concern for exercise. First, you want to be able to do more for longer periods, so you need to increase your tolerance for exertion. And you need to keep your muscles toned so you have the strength to do everyday tasks like bathing, dressing, and cooking.

Increasing your tolerance for exertion

Aerobic exercise — walking, swimming, step exercising, and riding a stationary bike — helps your lungs work better. Over time, you can increase not just how long or how often you exercise but how long and how often you can do other things. Most fitness experts recommend 30 minutes of aerobic exercise a day three to five times a week, but that's a general recommendation for generally healthy people. Your needs and abilities may be significantly different.

Where you start out in your exercise program is less important than the fact that you're starting to exercise. If you can only walk for three minutes or can only ride a stationary bike for a minute and a half before you feel short of breath, that's okay. The important thing is that you do what you can.

If you use oxygen, be sure to use it when you exercise, too (at the prescribed flow rate, of course). Your body requires more oxygen when you exercise, so keeping it on during your workout will help you feel more comfortable.

It's also important that you do what you can consistently. Three minutes of walking isn't helpful if you don't do it regularly; in fact, if you don't do it regularly, chances are it won't be long before you can't even go the three minutes. But if you make it a regular part of your routine, after a month or two you may be surprised at how long you can walk before stopping.

You're more likely to stick with your exercise plan if you choose an activity you enjoy, or at least one you don't dread. If you really don't care for riding a stationary bike, make walking, stair-stepping, or swimming your aerobic activity instead.

Walking

Walking is a popular exercise because it's cheap and can be done almost anywhere. If you can't walk very far at first, you can start by doing your daily walking at home; a few laps up and down your living room, for example, can fit easily and conveniently into your routine. As you get stronger and able to do more walking, you can go outdoors or, if weather or neighborhood conditions don't permit outdoor walking, check out your local shopping center. Many malls open early to accommodate walkers, especially when there's a local senior citizens walking group.

When you walk, do it slowly and carefully. Let your arms swing loosely, and take longer strides. **Remember:** You're not trying to catch a train; you're conditioning your lungs and body. Set a pace you're comfortable with and can keep up for a while — whether it's 3 minutes or 30.

Coordinate your breathing rhythm with your walking rhythm. Count how many steps you take when you inhale, and exhale for twice as many steps. If you walk three steps while you're breathing in, for example, you should exhale for six steps. This technique will help you pace yourself so your walking doesn't get ahead of your breathing.

Swimming

The term *swimming* may be a little misleading, because many COPD patients don't have enough lung function to do what we normally think of as actual swimming. But moving around in the water can be easier than moving around on land, and it's a relatively easy, gentle way to work your respiratory and circulatory systems. If you can't do regular swimming, walking laps around the shallow end of the pool may be a good alternative for you.

Aquatic exercise can also be the best option if you have joint problems; the buoyancy of the water relieves weight-bearing pressure on arthritic knees, for example, making it easier to get the exercise you need.

"Sneaky" aerobics

If you have a hard time sticking to a regular exercise schedule, you can try sneaking aerobic activity into your daily routine. Things like walking to work, to visit neighbors, or to do errands get you moving; walking the dog can benefit both you and your pet; even fast-paced sweeping or mopping can get your heart rate up.

There's an easy way to tell if you're exercising too hard, not hard enough, or at just the right pace. If you can sing while you're exercising, you're probably not working hard enough, but if you can't talk while you're exercising, you're probably working too hard. At the proper pace, you should be able to carry on a conversation while you're exercising.

Strengthening your limbs

Your arms and legs get weaker as you age, and those effects are often heightened by COPD. Strengthening exercises can help you keep the muscles in your upper and lower body toned so you feel more confident walking and lifting. You don't need any fancy equipment to do these exercises, but, as always, talk to your doctor before starting any strengthening program. He may have specific exercises to recommend, as well as guidelines on how often you should do them and how many repetitions you should aim for.

Upper-body exercises

Upper-body exercises tone the muscles in your shoulders and arms, which gives you more strength for things like carrying groceries or laundry, housework like dusting and sweeping or vacuuming, and lifting things like pots and pans when you're cooking. Toning your upper body also helps strengthen the muscles around your rib cage, and that can help make breathing easier.

Upper-body exercises are easy to do and don't require any special equipment. You can do them sitting on the edge of your bed, at your kitchen table, or while watching your favorite television program. Here are three to get you started:

- ✔ **Arm extensions:** This is just a matter of lifting your arm and holding it straight out from your body. Start with your arms at your side. As you exhale, raise one arm to the side until it's level with your shoulder. Hold it there for a second or two, then slowly bring it back down, inhaling as you do so. Alternate arms, and try to do a few repetitions for each arm.

- ✔ **Elbow breathing:** Sit up straight with your feet slightly apart. Put your hands flat on your chest with your fingertips touching and your elbows raised to about shoulder height. As you breathe in, pull your elbows back so your fingers are no longer touching. Exhale as you bring your elbows back to their original position and your fingertips touch again. Do this exercise slowly, and try to exhale for twice as long as you inhale.

- ✔ **Elbow circles:** Elbow circles can be done either sitting or standing. If you have difficulty with standing or keeping your balance, do this exercise sitting down with your feet slightly apart. Put your hands on your shoulders, with your elbows sticking out in front of you. Move your elbows in circles and concentrate on your breathing. You can inhale for one circle and exhale the next, or you can exhale as you begin the circle and inhale as you complete. Like the elbow breathing, this exercise should be done slowly so you can concentrate on taking deep breaths.

Lower-body exercises

The stronger your legs are, the easier it is for you to move around. You won't get tired as easily when you're standing, either, so you'll be able to move around for longer periods. Here are three good lower-body exercises:

- **Knee extensions:** Knee extensions help tone the muscles along the sides of your knee, as well as your thigh and calf muscles. You can do these exercises while watching TV or even reading. Just sit in a chair with your feet slightly apart. As you exhale, straighten your knee, raising your lower leg. Hold your leg out level with your hip for a second or two (longer if you can manage it); then breathe in as you bend your knee and bring your foot back to the floor. Alternate legs, and try to do a few repetitions with each leg.

- **Leg lifts:** Leg lifts are knee extensions extended, so to speak. When you do leg lifts, you straighten your knee and try to get your foot as far off the ground as you can, as if you're trying to touch your knee to your shoulder. As with the knee extensions, breathe out when you lift your leg and in as you bring it back down. Alternate legs, and try to do a few repetitions with each leg.

- **Stair stepping:** Stair stepping is another cheap, easy way to help strengthen your leg muscles. You don't need to use one of those intimidating machines in the gym, either; you can do it right in your own home. If you don't have stairs in your home, you can purchase a plastic platform designed for stepping exercise.

  To do stair stepping at home, stand at the foot of the stairs and hold onto the banister or railing with one hand. If you're using a platform, place it near a wall or counter — something you can hold onto to keep your balance. Then you just step up, left foot, right foot, and down, left foot, right foot. Do as many repetitions as you can before you feel short of breath.

Use slow and steady movements when you're stair stepping. Speed can make you lose your balance or trip and fall.

Warming up

Whether you do aerobic or strengthening exercises, you need to give your body time to warm up, to prepare for the additional exertion of exercise. If you're getting ready to do strengthening exercises, you can gently stretch your arms and legs before you start doing lifts and other exercises in earnest.

Don't get too intense with stretches before you exercise. Your muscles aren't as pliant as they will be after you're done exercising, so, to avoid injury, it's important to do only very gentle stretching as a warm-up to exercise.

Range-of-motion movements are a good way to warm up because they combine gentle stretching with actual movement. For your arms and shoulders, hold your arms straight out from your sides and make large, slow circles in the air with them; this loosens up the shoulder joints and prepares the arm muscles for more exertion.

For your legs, try very gentle lunges: Stand with your feet about shoulder-width apart and put one foot forward. Bend the knee of the forward leg and keep the back leg as straight as you can. Hold the stretch for a few seconds, then reverse legs.

Do lunges where you can hold onto something for balance, like a railing, chair, or counter. Put your leg only as far forward as you feel comfortable with; if you feel anything more than a slight taut sensation in your thigh or calf, bring your foot back toward your body a little.

If you're doing an aerobic activity like walking or water exercises, you can warm up by doing the activity at a slow pace for the first few minutes, then gradually increasing your pace as you get warmed up.

Cooling down

Depending on how long you exercise, your cooling down period should be five to ten minutes. This is when you keep moving your body (instead of stopping all movement abruptly) so your heart and breathing rate can gradually return to normal and so your muscles can gradually adjust to their resting state again.

Because your muscles are warm and flexible after exercise, this is an excellent time to do stretching. As with warming up, you don't want to overdo stretching during your cool down, but you probably will find it easier to stretch after exercise. You can do your stretches sitting or standing up.

Some simple cool-down moves include stretching your arms over your head, first one at a time and then together; stretching your arms straight out in front of you; and stretching your legs straight out, one at a time, and reaching your arms toward your outstretched foot. If you commonly have stiffness in your neck, you can stretch your neck muscles by moving your head in gentle circles. To stretch the muscles around your ribs, lean over to one side and then the other during your cool-down.

Skipping the cool-down phase — especially by sitting or lying down immediately after exercising — may make you feel dizzy or lightheaded. In some people, it can even cause heart palpitations. Just as it's easier on your body to gradually get up to your regular exercise rate, it's much less stressful to gradually reduce movement and exertion.

Designing Your Exercise Regimen

The first step in creating an exercise plan that works for you is to talk to your doctor. You need to discuss how much exercise you can or should do each day, how many days a week you should exercise, how your medications fit into your exercise plan, and what types of activities you should or should not do.

You also need to consider your own lifestyle and preferences. Some things to consider:

✔ Are you more likely to exercise on your own or with a buddy or group?

✔ What physical activities do you enjoy?

✔ Are there formal exercise programs that fit your needs?

✔ Are there limits on when, where, and how you can exercise?

For the last question, consider not just your physical health, but factors like getting to and from an exercise site, weather concerns (if any), and how participating in a more formalized program would fit into your schedule.

How to start

Sometimes starting any new routine is harder than actually doing it. And when you put off doing the things you know you should do, you may feel guilty or angry with yourself, and you get so busy dealing with those emotions that you end up putting off exercising even longer, which, in turn, makes you feel guiltier, and . . . well, you can see the pattern here.

Part of the problem with starting may be a sense of being overwhelmed. If you're thinking you need to start with 30 minutes a day, part of your brain says, "Whoa, no way." So reframe your thinking. You may want, eventually, to be able to do 30 minutes of exercise, but you certainly aren't going to start out that way.

Keep your initial goals small and reachable. That can mean different things depending on your circumstances. For your first exercise session, maybe your goal will be as simple as just doing it, or seeing how long you can do it. If all you can do to start is two or three minutes, that's fine; your goal then is to do those two or three minutes until you're comfortable enough to expand it to four or five minutes, and then to six or seven minutes, and so on.

Here are some other tips to help you get started:

✔ Choose a day to start exercising, and write it on your calendar.

✔ Choose a time when you have more energy; for many COPD patients, energy levels are highest in the mornings.

✔ Make sure you wait at least 90 minutes after a meal before you begin exercising; digestion takes a lot of energy, and you'll need it for exercising.

✔ Plan to exercise at the same time every day or every other day; write your schedule on your calendar as a reminder of your commitment.

✔ Write down how many minutes you exercise or how many repetitions you do each time; an exercise journal can help you track your progress.

✔ Allow yourself time to rest between exercising and other activities.

How often to do it

How often you exercise will depend on several factors, including how long you exercise at a time, how severe your COPD is, and your overall health. But, even if you can't do much at a time, you'll get more benefit from your exercise regimen if you do it regularly. There's nothing wrong with sporadic exercise; it's just that you don't get the cumulative benefits from now-and-then exercise.

You get the most benefit — and, thus, feel stronger and have less trouble with feeling short of breath — when exercise is a routine part of your schedule. Ideally, you should work up to doing 20 to 30 minutes of exercise three or four times a week.

Many people, both those with COPD and those who don't have any chronic health issues, find that exercising every other day works well for them. It becomes a regular part of your routine that way, but it also gives you days off so it doesn't fall into the drudgery category. Giving your body a full day to rest in between exercise sessions isn't a bad idea, either; you're less likely to be sore when your body has plenty of time to recover from exertion.

Even if you only exercise a few minutes at a time, you'll get the most benefit from it if you do it every other day. When you have COPD, the important thing is that you exercise regularly, not how much you can exercise.

How long to do it

The length of your exercise sessions depends on how healthy and fit you are to begin with. Talk to your doctor about reasonable goals for you. He likely will recommend starting with 10 or 15 minutes at a time — perhaps less if your situation calls for it — and gradually increasing the length of your workouts over several weeks or months.

You also can figure out how long you should be exercising in each session by listening to your body. If you feel sore, short of breath, or lightheaded, you should either cut back on the intensity of your workout or cut back on its length.

Your doctor or physical therapist may talk to you about the *RPE scale*. RPE stands for *rating of perceived exertion*, a fancy way of measuring how hard you think you're working when you exercise. The RPE scale runs from zero to ten and measures how easy or hard various activities are for you. At the low end would be things like sitting up in a chair, and at the high end would be things like running a mile or climbing several flights of stairs.

Generally, your exercise regimen should rate around a three or a four. You may find it moderately difficult, but it shouldn't be so difficult that you can't continue. On the other hand, if it's too easy, you probably aren't getting much benefit from it. When you're deciding where your exercise falls on the RPE scale, remember to take into account things like tightness or heaviness in your arms or legs as well as feeling short of breath.

When to take it easy

There are serious danger signs to watch out for when you're exercising:

- ✔ Excessive sweating
- ✔ Weakness, especially in the legs
- ✔ Chest pain
- ✔ Any kind of muscle pain
- ✔ Lightheadedness or dizziness

These are signs that you're overexerting yourself, and you should stop immediately and rest. If your breathing and heart rate don't return to normal in 15 to 20 minutes, call your doctor.

Pain is your body's early warning system to let you know that something's wrong. Never ignore pain; "working through it" can actually cause more damage and make the healing process much longer and more difficult.

You also should take it easy if you've been unusually active or tired in recent days. If you have a fever or any bout of illness, wait until you're fully recovered before resuming your exercise routine. If you get out of your routine for any significant length of time — say four days or more — lower the intensity and length of your exercise sessions until you feel confident and comfortable in resuming your normal levels.

If you usually exercise outdoors, pay attention to the weather. On days when it's very cold or very hot, avoid exercising outside; extremes in temperature can cause chest pain and difficulty breathing, as well as circulatory problems. High humidity also is a no-no when it comes to exercising, because it can make you tire more quickly.

Finally, check with your doctor about any effects your medications may have on your ability to exercise. Some meds can make you feel tired more easily, and some can change your body's response to any kind of exertion.

Part IV

Breathing Easier:
Living with COPD

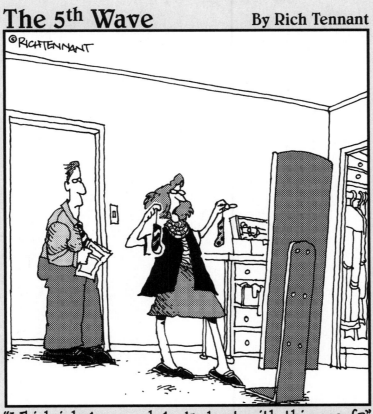

The 5th Wave   By Rich Tennant

"Which inhaler pouch looks best with this scarf?"

In this part . . .

COPD drains you of energy, making even the most mundane tasks exhausting. In this part, we break down the myriad ways COPD can affect your daily life, showing you why it can make routine activities more difficult and providing strategies for easing the strain. From the kind of clothing you choose to how you organize your kitchen, bath, bedroom, and living room, you can take practical steps to make your days less tiring and less stressful.

We also give you essential tips on preparing for those times when your symptoms are at their worst. We identify the danger signs that should alert you and your loved ones to get help right away, as well as the information you need when it's time to go to the emergency room.

In this part, we also devote an entire chapter to strategies on helping a loved one who has COPD.

Chapter 13

A Day in Your Life with COPD

*E*nergy is like money: It can be invested wisely, or it can be frittered away on things that aren't important. When you have COPD, you have to choose how you want to spend your energy and find ways to save your energy for the things that are most important to you.

That means, among other things, setting your priorities and identifying the best times to accomplish your priorities. This may require a little experimentation before you figure out when you usually have more energy and when you don't have much. It also may take you some time to figure out your limitations. This is common; most people have a mental picture of themselves and their abilities that is oddly capable of ignoring new conditions and realities. The result: They overextend themselves from time to time.

Another element in spending your energy wisely is finding ways to make things easier for yourself. In Chapter 14, we discuss ways to make your home easier for you to live in with COPD; in this chapter, we discuss ways to make your personal routine easier, from choosing comfortable clothing to adapting your work environment to getting out of the house.

As you live with COPD, you'll develop your own tricks and tips to help you make the most of your days. What we offer here are some suggestions to get you started — a list that is by no means comprehensive or universal. Feel free to discard or ignore the suggestions that don't make sense for you and to adapt any others so they work even better for you.

Your Daily Rhythm

In a typical 24 hours, your energy level will have peaks and valleys, and this is true whether you have COPD or not. The difference with COPD is that you have to pay closer attention to your unique daily rhythm and adapt your daily life to take advantage of both the high and low energy points. Your motto here is "Go with the flow," and "the flow" is your energy level.

Identifying your rhythm

Are you a morning person or an evening person? Many people with COPD find their energy levels are highest earlier in the day, possibly because they're coming off a good long rest. But that's by no means universal. Maybe your energy peaks at midday or later, and mornings are more of a gearing-up time for you.

It's important to figure out when you tend to be more (or less) energetic, because that critical piece of information can help you plan your day so you don't feel wiped out by the end of it. The better you are at organizing your routine around your energy cycles, the less likely you are to feel overwhelmed by your symptoms.

Here are some questions to help you decipher your own daily rhythm:

- ✔ Do you usually feel sluggish or energetic when you wake up in the morning?

- ✔ Are you more likely to sleep late in the morning or to get up early?

- ✔ If it were entirely up to you, would you rather stay up past midnight or go to bed before the 11 o'clock news?

- ✔ Would you rather do errands like grocery shopping in the morning or the afternoon?

- ✔ Do you take naps? If so, do you tend to nap more in the morning or in the afternoon?

After you've identified your body's rhythms, you can play with your daily routine so you can rest when you need to and get things done when you have the energy to do them.

Setting your priorities

Even the healthiest people don't always have the time or energy to do everything they'd like to do, and that can be even more frustrating when you have COPD. You may be inclined to fight against your limitations, but ignoring them won't make them go away, and the fight may leave you feeling even more drained, physically and emotionally.

Giving up certain things or activities may seem like an unwarranted sacrifice at first, but actually your COPD symptoms provide the perfect opportunity to decide what's really important to you. If you're like most people, there are probably a lot of things in your life — from physical items like furniture or collectibles to obligations of your time — that are there mainly because you've gotten accustomed to them being there, not because you have any particular attachment to them. This is your chance to identify the clutter in your life and do a good spring cleaning. You may be surprised at how much better you feel, especially mentally and emotionally, after you've cut out the things that mean the least to you.

Pacing yourself

Even after you've cleared your life of the things that don't matter to you much, you still may feel over-extended. This is where pacing comes in. Here are some dos and don'ts to help you organize your day:

- **Don't rush around.** Whenever possible, try to maintain a steady pace.

- **Don't set your expectations too high.** If anything, set the things you want to accomplish in the middling range; that way, you can do more if you have extra energy, and that can be a tremendous mental boost.

- **Don't try to do two high-energy things back to back.** Allow for a rest period in between tasks.

- **Don't try to do something immediately after eating.** Digestion takes a lot of your body's energy, so you should try to rest for at least 20 minutes after a meal — longer if you've had a big meal.

- **Do arrange your schedule so the most important things get done first.** Less important things can wait for another day if necessary.

- **Do ask family and friends for help, especially with tasks that require bending or lifting.**

- **Do use the most comfortable position for each thing you have to do.** Sitting takes less energy than standing, for example, so do as much as you can from a sitting position.

- **Do take advantage of your medications' benefits by planning to do important tasks right after taking your medicine, when you're likely to feel at your best.**

Morning rituals

For some people with COPD, just getting up and ready to face the day each morning can be a strain. Bathing, grooming, and getting dressed involve quite a bit of exertion, and you haven't even gotten to your to-do list yet. Fortunately, there are ways to minimize the drain on your limited energy.

Before you get out of bed

In your younger days, you may have leapt out of bed with a whoop and a holler every morning. But now you may find that you feel better if you take a less up-and-at-'em approach to starting your day. Those first few minutes after waking up are great for gently stretching your muscles and taking a few slow, deep breaths.

Your role model here is the typical house cat. Wiggle your fingers and toes, roll your shoulders, stretch your arms and legs, even yawn a time or two. Then, when it's time to sit up and take notice of the world around you, you can do it in a genteel, civilized way.

Washing up

Bathing can be an exhausting chore, but there are ways to make it easier. Sponge baths allow you to take your time over your ablutions, washing one area of your body at a time and resting as necessary. You also can sit down for most, if not all, of a sponge bath.

Standing in a shower takes more energy than sitting in a tub. However, because of the muscle weakness often associated with COPD, climbing in and out of a tub safely isn't always easy, either. One solution is to invest in a plastic shower chair that fits in the tub. Combined with a handheld shower head, this option allows you to sit comfortably while bathing and direct the water where you need it.

If you're using oxygen, drape your hose over the shower curtain rod to keep it out of your way while you're bathing.

Heat and humidity can make it harder to breathe. If you have an exhaust fan in your bathroom, always turn it on while you're bathing. If you don't have one, leave the bathroom door open least a little to allow the steam to escape. Lukewarm water doesn't produce as much steam as hot water, so you may find that it's easier to breathe with a not-quite-so-hot shower or bath.

Drying off after bathing can be difficult when you have COPD. Instead, buy a long terrycloth robe to wear when you get out of the shower or tub. It will absorb most of the water on your skin, and you can gently blot dry areas that are still wet.

General grooming

Using a chair at the bathroom sink can help you save energy while you wash your face, shave, brush your teeth, put on makeup, or comb your hair. Be sure to get a chair that puts you at a comfortable height for the sink, and get a small mirror for the vanity-top so you don't have to lean forward too much.

If you use oxygen, you can remove the cannula briefly to wash your face, shave, or put on makeup. Just make sure you pace yourself; if you get out of breath, put your cannula back on and rest until you feel better.

Aerosol sprays can make breathing harder, so try to avoid them, especially in the bathroom, where it's nearly impossible not to breathe in the spray. Use hair gel or mousse instead of hairspray and roll-on or stick deodorant instead of spray deodorant. When possible, get unscented varieties; the perfumes can hamper breathing, too.

Holding your arms up for any length of time can be quite tiring, so go for simple hairstyles that don't require a lot of blow-drying and styling.

Getting dressed

Putting your clothes together before you start getting dressed can save you a lot of unnecessary movement. When you first get up in the morning, for example, have your robe and slippers within easy reach of the edge of the bed so you can put them on while you're sitting.

When you're ready to get dressed for the day, get all the items you're going to wear together so you don't have to move around the room to put on each garment. Then sit on a chair or the bed and take your time getting dressed; rushing will take more energy and may make you feel anxious, which can lead to breathing problems.

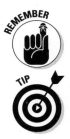

Your goal is to minimize movement, so try little tricks like placing your underwear inside your slacks and pulling them on together.

Dressing the lower part of your body takes more energy, so start with your feet and work your way up. Reaching tools can help you pull on socks without having to bend over; if you don't have one of these tools or you don't like to use them, lift your feet to you. A footstool next to the bed can support your feet and legs while you're putting on socks, underwear, and pants.

Energy for the afternoon

Many people, even those without COPD, seem to fall into an energy slump around midafternoon. Some cultures deal with this phenomenon with the post-lunch nap or rest period; before the days of globalization, for example, most businesses in places like Greece were traditionally closed for a few hours in the afternoon.

Many people who have COPD find their energy levels falling way below par in the afternoon. Sometimes this is because they've been unusually active in the morning; more often, though, it's just part of their normal energy rhythm.

Rest and pacing are the keys to maintaining some level of energy throughout the day. Build frequent rest breaks into your daily routine; try to rest for at least a few minutes in between each activity. Resting is particularly important after eating because digestion takes a lot of energy.

If you're able to take one, you may find that a brief nap in the afternoon helps recharge your batteries.

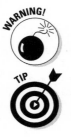

Don't lie down immediately after eating. Your full stomach can put additional pressure on your lungs when you lie down, making breathing more difficult. Rest sitting up in a comfortable chair for at least 20 minutes after meals.

Try to arrange your schedule so you can do less energy-consuming tasks in the afternoon. This may be the time for you to do quiet chores like balancing the checkbook or organizing things to be filed.

Quiet evenings

By the time evening rolls around, many people with COPD find that all they really want to do is sit down and relax. If you've been accustomed to activity-filled evenings, this can be a hard adjustment to make; giving up things you used to enjoy, like volunteer meetings or outings with friends, can present significant emotional and mental challenges.

Depending on how severe your COPD is and how flexible your schedule is, you may be able to find ways to continue doing those sorts of things, though on a smaller scale. Maybe you can do a few hours of volunteer work on Saturday mornings instead of Tuesday evenings, for example. Instead of planning to go out to dinner with friends on a Friday night, maybe you can get together for Sunday brunch.

Unless you get your second wind, so to speak, after dinner, you'll probably feel better if you generally leave your evenings free from various obligations. Knowing you can rest tonight can help you find the energy you need to do something this morning.

When you do have some evening obligation, try to arrange your schedule so you can rest up for it during the day and recover from it the next day. Don't plan to do anything taxing that morning or the next; you may feel more tired than usual the day after an evening outing, and an extra 24 hours of "light duty" can help you restore your normal energy levels.

Finally, get ready for bed in stages. Taking an hour or even half an hour to unwind can help you reduce anxiety and sleep better so you feel more rested when you wake up. Try changing into your pajamas and robe, then watch a favorite TV show before you go in to brush your teeth and wash your face. Read a few pages of a good book, either in your favorite chair or sitting up in bed before you turn the light out. Practice your deep breathing exercises in the dark, and let sleep come to you naturally.

Loosening Up

Choosing the right clothing can be tricky when you have COPD. Not only are tight, constricting garments uncomfortable, but they can make breathing feel even more difficult than it already is. This doesn't mean you're doomed to wear muumuus and sweatpants for the rest of your life (not that there's anything wrong with that if your tastes run that way), but it may mean you have to put more thought into your wardrobe than you're used to.

Starting from the foundations

For women, bras, panties, and other underclothing can present difficulties. Girdles, long out of fashion except for older generations, and corsets — now, inexplicably, regaining favor in the fashion world — are particularly nasty culprits, as are pantyhose and socks or stockings with overly binding tops.

Fortunately, you have several options. You can simply forego any kind of bra, for instance. If you aren't comfortable doing that, you can switch to sports bras, which offer support without biting into your shoulders or torso. Camisoles are another option; many are made to be worn visibly under a jacket or sweater, so you can be comfortable and fashionable at the same time.

Avoid panties that have "tummy control" features, because they can make you feel restricted in your breathing. Instead, choose cotton briefs that fit properly — that is, ones that don't cut into your waist too tightly or bind around your hips. Some women find that the new "boy shorts" design, a modified boxer style, offers the most comfort and freedom of movement.

Cotton is the best choice for underwear because it reduces chafing, especially in hot, humid conditions. It's usually more comfortable throughout the day than nylon or other fabrics, too.

Men should keep the same things in mind when choosing underwear. Whether you prefer boxers or briefs, make sure you wear the right size so the elastic waistband (and, in the case of briefs, the binding around the legs) fits comfortably. If you wear undershirts, V-necks may be the better choice; the necklines on crewneck shirts can be uncomfortable and even interfere with breathing if they're too tight.

Pantyhose are no longer de rigueur for women, which is a good thing when you have COPD. Not only can they be terribly uncomfortable, but they can be especially difficult to put on when you have breathing problems. If you shrink from showing your bare legs, consider wearing knee- or thigh-high hose or trouser socks; just make sure the elastic tops don't bind your legs.

Choosing the right clothes and accessories

Buttons, snaps, laces, and such can be real energy-stealers when you're trying to get dressed, especially if you suffer from arthritis or have trembling in your hands. Pull-on pants and skirts with elastic waists (properly fitted so the waist isn't too tight, of course) are easier to put on than ones with lots of buttons and zippers and whatnot. It's easier, too, to pull on a shirt or blouse than to struggle with half a dozen buttons or a zipper in the back. Men who have to wear button-down shirts for work or social engagements can save themselves some energy by buttoning all but the top two or three buttons beforehand and pulling the shirt on over their heads.

Freedom for your neck

Tight collars and neckties are a COPD no-no; fortunately, fashions for men, even in professional settings, have gotten more casual, so it's usually acceptable to wear an open collar with a very loosely tied tie or even no tie at all. If you must wear a tie, leave the top button of your shirt unbuttoned and adjust the tie knot so that it rests lightly at the base of your throat, not snug against your neck.

"Choker" necklaces are popular for women, but you should avoid them when you have COPD. If you like to wear necklaces, choose longer pendants or chains that don't constrict your neck.

Freedom for your waist

Belts can constrict the abdomen, so it's harder to expand your tummy when you're taking in a breath. Women can use scarves or woven belts, loosely tied or wrapped around the waist. Men may find that suspenders are more comfortable; with all the fun colors and designs available these days, they even add a dash of panache to the male wardrobe.

Freedom for your feet

Comfortable shoes are essential when you have COPD. High heels can cause balance problems if you have any symptoms of muscle weakness, not to mention pain in the toes, arches, and ankles. Slip-on, flat-heeled shoes are the best option when you have COPD: They're easy to put on, they support your feet, and they give you more stability when you're walking. There are lots of styles available, too, so you can still be fashionable. And now that sneakers with hook-and-loop closures are so common, you may never have to bend over to tie your shoes again.

A long-handled shoe horn can make it a lot easier to put your shoes on. Your local drugstore may carry one with a 12- to 18-inch handle. If you can't find one there, ask the pharmacist if one can be ordered for you or search online.

Dressing for the weather

Loose and light are the key words when it comes to coats and jackets. Wearing a heavy coat can put the same strain on you as carrying a heavy bag, and a coat that's too tight may restrict your breathing. For women, capes and swing coats are fashionable alternatives and, depending on the material they're made of, have the advantage of being both light and roomy. For men, car-length jackets may prove easier to wear and move around in than bulky long coats.

Like your shoes, boots should be comfortable and easy to put on. Flat heels provide better walking stability, especially in wet or icy conditions, than wedge or high heels. Choose a boot with a good tread to give you grip on uneven or slick surfaces.

A lightweight scarf can provide surprising warmth around your neck or ears, and, if necessary, you can put it over your nose and mouth to help warm the air before you breathe in.

Running Hot and Cold

Sometimes COPD can make you much more sensitive to heat and cold. Exceptionally hot or cold air can make it harder to catch your breath, and you may find that your comfort range has narrowed significantly as your COPD has progressed. Fortunately, you can use all kinds of tricks to stay in, or at least near, your comfort zone.

Fans and air-conditioning

When the weather is hot and humid, it can feel like a heavy blanket pressing down on your entire body. Expanding your chest and abdomen to breathe in becomes harder, and, if it's really humid, you may feel like you're trying to inhale fog instead of air.

Strategically placed fans can help by keeping the air moving. Ceiling fans are a good option for circulating air throughout the room, but sometimes they don't do enough to get you back in your comfort zone. For those times, you may want to have an oscillating fan near you; they're available in both table-top and floor models. Oscillating fans are preferable to stationary fans because they circulate the air in your immediate area instead of blowing constantly in one direction.

Fans can blow dust and other particles into the air, either from nearby furniture or from its own blades. Make sure the furniture around you is clean, and periodically wash (or have a family member, friend, or home aide do so) the fan blades and protective covering.

Air conditioners cool the air by removing the moisture from it, and they're particularly useful when the air outside is full of dust, pollen, ozone, or other irritants. If you don't have central air conditioning in your home, invest in one or two window units. They are relatively inexpensive, and the newer models are energy-efficient so your electricity bills won't shoot through the roof. It's a good idea to have at least two: one for the bedroom, and one for the room where you spend most of your waking hours at home. Even if you can't cool the rest of the house, you'll have a room or two to escape to if the heat and humidity are too much for you.

Continually moving from a hot environment to a cold one can cause headaches and other symptoms, so try to keep your trips between extreme temperatures at a minimum. Set your air conditioner at a reasonable temperature — between 68°F and 72°F (20°C–22°C) for most people — and resist the urge to overcompensate for the heat by "super-cooling" with air conditioning. Very often, after sitting quietly for a few minutes in a cool (not cold) area, feelings of being overheated will subside.

Heating options

Heating your home can pose some real challenges when you have COPD. Solid-fuel heating systems — those that use fuel oil, propane, kerosene, or wood — can give off fumes and particles that make it harder to breathe. Furnace maintenance is important, too, because dirty filters or ducts can fill your home's air with tiny airborne particles.

Here are some things to keep in mind about heating your home:

- ✔ Use high-quality filters in your furnace.
- ✔ Change your furnace filters regularly — every 30 to 90 days, depending on the type.
- ✔ Have your furnace cleaned and checked every fall to make sure it's working efficiently.
- ✔ Install carbon monoxide detectors in your home and change the batteries every six months.
- ✔ Make sure your doors and windows are caulked and weather-stripped to reduce drafts.

Don't cover your windows with plastic to keep drafts out during the winter. This technique can trap dangerous fumes and gases, including carbon monoxide, in your home. Instead, invest in insulated curtains or drapes to help minimize drafts.

Space heaters

In the winter, being too cold is the problem. If your home is drafty or poorly insulated, there may be areas of your house that are colder than others, and space heaters may make sense for you. Keep in mind, however, that, unlike humans, space heaters are not created equal.

Kerosene and propane heaters are *not* recommended when you have COPD. Not only do they pose a fire hazard — and, if you're using oxygen, anything that poses a fire hazard is a *big* concern — but the fumes they emit can make breathing even more difficult for you.

Electric space heaters are a much more sensible option. They're more convenient: You don't have to worry about running out of fuel. They're compact, so they don't get in your way. Many of them are programmable, so you can set them to turn on and off at specific times. Most of them have safety sensors so they automatically shut off if they're tipped over. And, like newer air conditioners, the newer electric space heaters are energy-efficient, so they don't cost that much to run.

No matter what kind of space heater you use, be sure to place it well away from other furniture, curtains, and anything else that may pose a fire risk. In particular, make sure your oxygen hose *never* comes in contact with the heater.

If you use a kerosene or propane heater, place the unit near a window and open the window a crack to allow the fumes to escape.

Blankets and throws

A simple, cost-effective way to stay warm is to have several lightweight blankets placed around your home so you can cover up easily if you get chilly. When you don't need them, they can be draped artistically over the corner of a chair or couch or folded up and placed on a footstool or in a convenient drawer.

Shawls are easier to put on and take off than sweaters or sweatshirts, and they do a good job of keeping your upper body warm.

 Use an electric blanket on your bed. They're lightweight, and most of them have thermostats so you can set the heat at a level that's comfortable for you. Unless you live in a very cold climate, you may find that you don't need any other blankets to sleep comfortably during the winter.

Working with COPD

COPD is the second-leading cause of disability in the United States. Few people with severe COPD work at all, and even moderate COPD can force you to scale back from a full-time job to a part-time one.

Whether you can keep working with COPD depends on a number of factors beyond the severity of your symptoms. If your job requires a lot of physical exertion, chances are, you'll have to either cut back or switch jobs if you want to keep working. Sedentary jobs that involve lots of sitting and very little lifting, bending, standing, or walking are easier to do when you have COPD, although it still can take a lot out of you. Some people find that their powers of concentration are less dependable, too.

If you want to continue working, you'll probably have to make the same kinds of adjustments in your routine on the job that you make in your routine at home. Your goal is to do what you can to lessen the strain that your job puts on you, while giving your employer the productivity she needs.

Talking to your employer

If your doctor okays you to continue working, he may put some restrictions on the type of work you can do. In that case, you'll have to discuss options with your employer. Depending on your relationship with your employer, you may want to consult an attorney who specializes in employment law. No one likes to think an employer would act unethically or illegally when a worker discloses that he has COPD, but the reality is that people do lose their jobs for all kinds of reasons, some of them unfair and some of them against the law. An employment law attorney can tell you what protections you have, which may vary significantly from state to state.

Adjusting your duties

Changing your job description to eliminate duties that cause problems for you may be possible. You'll have to negotiate any such changes with your employer, of course. Before you go into your boss's office to discuss this, think about alternatives for getting the job done even if you can no longer do all the things you have been doing in your position. You can ease much of your boss's understandable anxiety by presenting possible solutions to the problem.

Don't know where to start? Here are some things to consider:

- **Is there anyone else who can do the tasks I can't do anymore?** If part of your job calls for lifting heavy objects, maybe someone else in your workplace could take over that task for you. In return, perhaps you could take on some of that person's workload.

- **Are there tools or devices that will permit me to continue those tasks?** There may be ways to make difficult tasks easier at work. You can use wheeled tables and hand carts to move around heavy things; ramps may make it easier to move things from one level to another.

- **Can my workspace be rearranged to minimize difficult tasks?** Maybe you can organize your desk or work area differently so you don't have to bend, reach, or lift so much. If you're used to standing while you do your work, a simple change like a stool that you can sit or lean on may allow you to continue working.

- **Are there openings in less strenuous positions that I would be qualified for?** If it isn't practical for you to work on the factory floor any more, perhaps you could change to a desk job that doesn't require as much physical exertion.

Adjusting your schedule

Depending on the severity of your COPD and how it progresses, you may not have the energy to put in a full workday every day, or you may need longer break periods to re-energize. Perhaps you can cut back your hours or work from home one or two days a week. You may be able to work out a flex-time schedule so you can come in later in the morning, take longer lunch breaks, or even take a long afternoon break when your energy level is at its lowest.

Even if your boss is the kindest and most compassionate person you know, he still has to keep the welfare of the business in mind. Flex time may not meet your employer's needs, and some jobs — retail, factory work, and the like — cannot be performed from home. Don't be shy about talking about your needs, but remember that your employer may not have the flexibility you'd like.

Knowing when you shouldn't work

If your job exposes you to secondhand smoke, chemical fumes, dust, or other forms of airborne irritants, your doctor likely will recommend that you switch jobs. All these things can make your COPD much worse much faster, and your doctor's goal is to keep you as healthy as possible for as long as possible.

There are other times when you shouldn't work. If you have a respiratory infection or other acute illness, the best thing you can do for yourself is stay home and rest. If there's a bug going around the office, you may want to keep your distance, too; when you have COPD, you're more susceptible to all kinds of contagious illnesses, especially colds, flu, and pneumonia.

You shouldn't force yourself to go to work when you're feeling exceptionally tired or weak. "Shaking it off" and "playing through the pain" may be laudable in sports, but ignoring your body's signals can lead to serious problems when you have COPD. If you're tired and weak, it's most likely because your body isn't getting enough oxygen. Additional stress — like forcing yourself to move when you really don't have the energy — can prompt acute exacerbations of your symptoms, so you end up feeling worse than you did before.

Planning for a time when you can't work

As we mentioned at the beginning of this section, COPD is one of the most common reasons people become unable to work at all. It can be quite a blow when your doctor says you shouldn't work; for many people, a big chunk of their identity and sense of self-worth is wrapped up in their chosen occupations. And that doesn't even take into account the financial issues so many people have to grapple with when they become disabled.

Because COPD so often leads to permanent disability, it makes sense for you to plan ahead for the day when you'll no longer be able to work. In the following sections, we cover some things you need to consider.

How will you survive financially?

Check your employer's benefit package to find out if disability benefits are included, how long they last, and what's required to qualify for them. Most disability plans pay between 50 percent and 60 percent of your gross wages; in many cases, if you contribute to the cost of the disability insurance, your income benefits from the policy are not taxable (check with your accountant or financial planner to find out the tax rules in your state). Also look into what it takes to receive Social Security disability benefits. You can get basic information at the Social Security Administration's Web site (www.ssa.gov); its Benefit Eligibility Screening Tool, which takes only a few minutes to complete, can help you identify the benefits you may qualify for. The Disability Planner section provides information on how to qualify and apply for benefits, and a benefit calculator gives you a rough idea of how much you can expect to receive in monthly benefits.

It can take two years or more to have your Social Security Disability Insurance application approved, and many employer-paid disability insurance plans pay benefits for only six months or less. You'll need a financial plan to see you through the gap in benefits, so consulting a professional financial planner is wise.

If you don't already have your own disability insurance policy, you may not be able to find an affordable one after you've been diagnosed with COPD because it's considered a preexisting condition, which most policies won't cover. Even if you could find an insurer to write a policy that doesn't exclude your COPD, the premiums likely would be astronomical.

How will your medical bills be paid?

Now is the time to find out whether your employer's insurance will cover your doctor bills, prescriptions, and hospitalizations if you have to go out on disability. Also find out how long you'll have any coverage so you don't get any nasty surprises from that quarter down the road.

How will you feel mentally and emotionally when you can't work?

Depression is common among unemployed people, regardless of the cause for the unemployment. Some retirees even have a hard time adjusting to a life where work is no longer part of the equation. By assessing your feelings about not working — and especially not being *able* to work — before that day comes, you're better prepared to deal with your own emotional responses when it does arrive.

How will your family and friends feel when you can't work?

Going out on disability can be as tough on your loved ones as it is on you, although in different ways. It's hard to see someone you love unable to do the things he used to do, and it's hard to adjust your mental image of that person to the new reality. Talking about it before it happens can help alleviate the shock, grief, and sense of helplessness that loved ones often experience when your health puts severe limits on your activities.

Outings with COPD

You may have COPD, but that doesn't mean you have to be housebound day in and day out. Even if you're on oxygen therapy, you can get out and about when you feel up to it, as long as you're smart about what you do and when you do it.

Choosing your activities

At the beginning of this chapter, we likened energy to money — a limited resource to be invested wisely. This is especially true when it comes to deciding what you want to do outside your home. You probably don't have enough energy to do everything you used to do or would like to do, so you have to choose the activities that are most important to you — the ones you really want to invest your energy in.

As with your daily routines at home and, when it applies, at work, choosing your activities is a matter of setting your priorities. If you really want to get together with your canasta group Tuesday afternoon, you'll probably have to turn down going to the movies on Monday and put off your regular Wednesday trip to the grocery store until Thursday.

Knowing your limits

One thing COPD teaches you pretty fast is how to read the signals your body sends you. It's important to pay attention to those signals and respond accordingly. Don't let guilt or stubbornness prevent you from taking proper care of yourself. Instead, think of it along the lines of "living to fight another day." If you respect your limits, you'll have fewer episodes where your symptoms are severe enough to keep you from doing anything, so you'll be able to do some things more often.

Knowing your limits is really the art of compromise. Maybe you don't have the energy to stay up until midnight on New Year's Eve to see the ball drop in Times Square. But you may be able to attend your neighbor's New Year's Eve party for an hour or so earlier in the evening. If you're too tired to cope with going to a movie theater, you can wait until the movie comes out on video or DVD, rent it, and watch it with family or friends in the comfort of your home.

Saying no (gracefully)

When you have COPD, you have to allow yourself to say no to invitations when you just don't feel up to going out. *Remember:* You're the only one who really knows how you feel, so you're the only one who can decide whether you have the energy to do something. Friends and family may be disappointed if you don't have the energy to go out with them, but they'll understand. You should never let yourself succumb to guilt for having to turn down an invitation.

In the same vein, COPD provides the perfect excuse to get out of doing things you *don't* want to do without being impolite or hurting anybody's feelings. Invited to dinner at a bore's house? "I'd love to, but I just don't have the energy to get out much anymore. Thanks so much for inviting me, though."

Checking the weather

Nearly everyone keeps an eye on the weather when they're planning a picnic, a camping or fishing trip, or even a long drive to spend the holidays with friends or relatives. But when you have COPD, the weather is a critical variable in your plans. Hot and humid weather can exacerbate your breathing difficulties; so can very cold weather. Air pollution, smog alerts, and ozone warnings are all signs that you should stay indoors as much as possible. Cold, rainy days may overwhelm your immune system (your body diverts more energy to staying warm, which can weaken your immune system) and make you more susceptible to colds, chills, and fever.

Unless it's absolutely necessary, you should avoid going out when the weather is extreme. Depending on where you live, this may sound like house arrest; after all, the weather is seldom ideal every day, and sometimes it's not even ideal on most days. The key really is, again, knowing your limits and, when you do go out, dressing appropriately for the conditions.

Planning ahead

Good planning covers both your outing and your return home. You want to make things as easy as you can for yourself in both instances. With enough planning (and your doctor's permission, if your health status warrants it), you can even take vacations with COPD.

Going to the grocery store, the post office, the bank, or the dry cleaner can be exhausting no matter how good your health is. When you have COPD, just the thought of doing these typical errands can make you feel tired. But there are ways to minimize the drain on your energy levels.

For shopping trips:

- ✔ **Choose a time when the stores are less likely to be crowded.** Mornings in the middle of the week are usually best.
- ✔ **Make a list of the stores you want to visit and what you want to shop for at each one.**
- ✔ **For your grocery list, put items in the order you'll find them in the store so you don't have to retrace your steps.**
- ✔ **If the store you're going to has carts, use one.** It provides support while you walk and you can put your purse or portable oxygen tank in it.

Depending on how severe your COPD is and other health factors, you may qualify for a handicapped parking permit. Ask your doctor how to apply for one, and, if you do qualify, use it; saving a few steps in the parking lot means more energy for completing your errands.

For social outings:

- ✔ **Try to schedule your social engagements for the time of day when you feel most energetic.**
- ✔ **Make the time to rest before you go out.**
- ✔ **Schedule your get-together around your medication schedule if possible.** If you're supposed to take a nebulizer treatment at 3 o'clock, plan to be home by then.
- ✔ **Take your portable medications — pills, inhalers, and so on — with you.**

Always, always, always carry your rescue inhaler with you, no matter where you go. It's your first line of defense for acute exacerbations.

✔ If you're eating out, choose light fare from the menu, or ask for your meal to be split in two and take half home with you.

✔ Plan to take it easy after you get home.

For overnight and longer trips:

✔ If you're on oxygen, make sure you have plenty to last for your trip.

✔ If you're traveling by air, make arrangements with the airline regarding your oxygen.

✔ Take enough of your medications to get you through your trip, along with extra doses in case you're delayed getting home.

✔ Try to avoid driving or taking public transportation during rush hours.

✔ If you're driving or riding in a car, schedule frequent rest stops so you can get out and stretch your limbs.

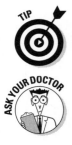

If you have to pump gas into your car yourself, try to stand upwind from the pump handle to avoid inhaling gas fumes. You may also cover your nose and mouth with a scarf or handkerchief to minimize the odds of inhaling noxious fumes.

Share your travel plans with your doctor, and ask if she has any advice or concerns. For instance, you may not have to use your oxygen on a plane once it reaches cruising altitude; your doctor can tell you. Also, if you're going someplace that's at a significantly different altitude, your doctor may give you different instructions for using oxygen and even taking your meds.

To prepare for your return home (no matter how long you'll be gone):

✔ Lay your pajamas and robe or other loungewear out on the bed so you can change into comfortable clothes as soon as you want to.

✔ If possible, prepare your next round of medications and leave them ready on the table or counter.

✔ Have a meal or snack already made so you don't have to make it when you get home.

✔ If you'll be returning after sunset, leave the porch light on outside and a lamp on inside so you don't have to grope in the dark.

✔ Give yourself permission to put off household chores, even if only for today. The dirty dishes in the sink can wait until morning, just this once.

In addition to emergency contact information, carry a list of your medications, including the dose and frequency, and the name and phone number of your doctor in your wallet. This will be of immense help to medical personnel if you need emergency medical care when you're away from home.

Chapter 14

Making Your Home You-Friendly

COPD interferes with the body's ability to receive and distribute oxygen, and that can turn even the most routine household activities into honest-to-goodness chores. You may feel dizzy or lightheaded when you bend over or stand up. The exertion of walking even a few feet may leave you short of breath. You may feel too weak to lift things above your chest. And the less you feel able to do, the more likely you are to feel discouraged and depressed.

Making adjustments around your home can help you ward off those bad feelings. When it's easier to get through your day, you enjoy a sense of independence — and that's one of the best antidotes to depression.

Just *thinking* of changing your home to meet your needs as a COPD sufferer can be daunting. You may feel a sense of loss because you can't do things the way you've always done them. You may feel like you're stuck with the way things are arranged now. Or you may feel awkward about asking everyone in your household to accommodate *your* needs. All these feelings are normal.

But these feelings also have their flip sides. You've changed the way you do things many times to accommodate other changes in your life — when you and your partner got together, for example, or when your children came along, or when one of you changed jobs, or when you moved to a new house or city. So you know how to make changes that make sense for you, and in many ways, this is just another one of those situations where changes make sense.

Asking others in your home to deal with changes may seem like an unreasonable demand, but the truth is that, by making these changes, you're reducing your dependence on your family members. When things are arranged so that you can do certain tasks yourself, you boost your own self-esteem and give your loved ones more freedom to do other things.

Making your home more user-friendly can be a challenge, and you may have to get creative to find ways around the unique obstacles in your home. In this chapter, we show you ways to reorganize your living space to make things more convenient for you, and we talk about tools and accessories that can help you in your reorganization. We also offer tips for simplifying your daily routine and delegating energy-draining tasks to others. The information in this chapter will empower you to make these changes, and it may even make you eager to get started!

It's All within Reach

When you have COPD, you may have a hard time lifting, carrying, bending, and stretching, and those limitations make a lot of daily activities much more difficult. Even something as simple as pulling up the covers on your bed can be an exhausting feat.

Because you have COPD, your body has to work harder to distribute oxygen. Every time you move, you use up energy your body needs to keep breathing.

Fortunately, you can do many things to make your daily routine more convenient and easier on your body.

Reorganizing things you use often

Ideally, everything you need in your home would be handily stored in drawers or on shelves located somewhere between your waist-level and your shoulder-level. This setup would make everything easy to get to whether you were standing, sitting, or lying down.

Real life often isn't ideal, though, and if you're like most people, you have way more stuff than can fit into that ideal waist-level-to-shoulder-level space. So the trick is to identify what you use the most and figure out how to organize that stuff so it's readily accessible.

Ask family members or friends for help in reorganizing. Having help will make the task easier on you, and they'll be delighted at the opportunity to provide practical assistance.

When you start thinking of rearranging your entire home, you can easily become overwhelmed, so don't think of it that way. Instead, break the job down room by room.

One tip that applies to the whole house: Because your body uses so much energy to breathe, there's not a lot left over to help you move. So keeping your home free of clutter and obstacles is important. If you have to zig and zag around furniture, you may be better off getting rid of a few nonessential pieces or rearranging them so you have clear walkways in each room. The wider the traffic paths through your home, the better — especially if you're using oxygen and have to roll a tank with you or trail a line to your stationary concentrator. Look for places where turns are difficult or your line tends to get caught, and see if you can eliminate or minimize those hazards.

In the bedroom

The nightstand by your bed should have a telephone, a clock, and a lamp with a switch that's easy to locate. You may also want to keep a bottle or glass of water on your nightstand if you tend to wake in the middle of the night with a cough, a dry feeling in your mouth, or a tickle in your throat — all common symptoms for people using oxygen. If you take medications right before bed, you may want to keep the meds on your nightstand, too.

Having a bench or chair in your bedroom is a good idea. You can use it to lay out your clothes for the day or your pajamas and robe for the night. You also can use it to sit on while you get dressed and undressed. A footstool is handy to use when you're putting on socks and shoes, too.

Arrange your dresser drawers so that the clothes you wear most often are in the upper drawers. This will help you avoid a lot of bending and tugging at drawers. In your closet, use the shelf above the rod to store rarely used items. If you need shelf space to store things you use regularly, look into installing vertical shelves; that way, you'll have two or three shelves at a comfortable height and won't have to exert yourself by stretching and pulling things down from above.

In the bathroom

Bending or crouching to rummage through things under the bathroom sink can be uncomfortable when you have COPD. A better option is to use shelves and storage units designed for bathrooms to keep essential items within easy reach. You can minimize clutter by using baskets to hold things like makeup, hairbrushes, blow dryers, and so on. Many home-improvement stores carry slimmed-down drawer units that fit between the vanity and toilet; these can be useful for storing things like hand towels, soaps, toilet paper, and first-aid kits.

Consider using a stool or chair in front of the sink when you brush your teeth and wash your face; sitting takes less energy than standing does. If you can't see yourself in the mirror from a sitting position, put a small stand-up mirror on the counter when you shave, put on makeup, or fix your hair. You can also use the chair to lay out clothes or your towel when you bathe.

You may want to put a waterproof chair in your tub or shower so you can sit while you bathe. A handheld shower hose and head can make bathing easier, too, because you can direct the water where you want it. Use wire shelving designed to hang from the shower head or suction-cup baskets that attach to the tile to keep bath items together and in easy reach. Smaller bottles of shampoo, conditioner, and body wash are easier to grip than large bottles; you can buy plastic travel bottles, label them with a waterproof marker, and refill them as needed. An added bonus: They don't take up as much space in the shower or tub.

In the kitchen

The kitchen can be the most difficult room to organize, even if you don't have COPD. The trick here is to keep within easy reach the things you use most often. That means, for example, storing plates, bowls, cups, and glasses on the bottom shelves of your wall cabinets so you don't have to stretch too far to get to them. If you have room, store a frying pan, a sauce pan, and a baking dish there, too; that way you won't have to bend over to get these things out of your under-counter cabinets as often.

Slide-out trays and baskets for your under-counter cabinets make it easier to see what you've got and reach it. Lazy Susans are excellent additions to pantries and cabinets, because they allow you to see spices, storage containers, and various other sundries with just a spin.

Keep a tall stool in the kitchen so you can sit at the counter while you prepare foods or at the sink while you wash up.

Eliminate unnecessary movement around the kitchen by keeping like things together. Use a decorative canister to store coffee on the countertop next to the coffeemaker, for example, and keep your coffee cups in the cabinet above (on the bottom shelf, naturally). You can keep coffee filters in a drawer underneath the coffeemaker or on top of your coffee cups, so everything is right where you need it.

The same principle applies to organizing your pantry, freezer, and refrigerator. Keep like things together: sugar, flour, and other staples grouped together, canned goods together, and so on. Put the things you use most often on the middle shelves so you can easily see and reach them. Things you don't use as often can go on top or bottom shelves.

In the living room

The living room is most likely where you spend much of your time; it's a natural place for reading, watching television, visiting with family and friends, and generally relaxing. You need a comfortable place to sit, a table large enough to hold the things you want to have near you, and good lighting for reading and other hobbies like needlework or knitting.

Choosing "your" place to sit, whether it's an easy chair or a corner of the couch, is no small matter. You need a chair that fits your body and doesn't interfere with breathing:

- **The headrest should not push your head forward.** If your head is pushed forward, that puts strain on your neck muscles and can make breathing more difficult.

- **The chair should have lumbar support.** The *lumbar region* is your lower back, and a chair with lumbar support eases pressure on your lower back and allows your diaphragm to expand as needed.

- **You should be able to bend your knees comfortably over the edge of the seat while still having good support from the back, without having to slouch.** Slouching can make breathing more difficult.

Your end table should be spacious enough to keep the things you need within easy reach. If you use a nebulizer, you may want to keep it on the table so you can watch TV or read during your treatments. You'll probably want a box of tissues there, too, along with room for a glass of water and perhaps the book you're reading, the TV remote, and a telephone so you don't have to get up to make or answer calls. You may even want to keep your medications on this table; you can use pillboxes or a basket to keep them from taking over the table's surface.

Lighting should be strong enough so that you don't have to strain to read, and the switch should be handy to you in a seated position. If you prefer a floor lamp, position it so you can reach the switch without having to contort your body or get up from your seat.

One final thing you should have in your living room: a clock that you can see clearly. This is especially important if you're taking timed medications. Don't rely on the clock on your cable box; get a wall clock or an alarm clock with a battery backup. That way, even if the power goes out or a plug gets pulled out of the outlet, you'll always know what time it is.

Laundry room

Put your front-load washer and dryer on blocks or purchase one of the new storage base units so you don't have to bend to get clothes in or out. (If you have a top-load washer, putting it on blocks will make it harder for you to reach the bottom of the basket, unless you're exceptionally tall.) Set up a table with a chair so you can sit while you sort or fold clothes. If you iron, do it while sitting down, and invest in an asbestos pad so you don't have to stand the iron up each time. Install a tension-pole hangar rack near the washer and dryer (or ironing board) so you can hang clothes easily. A wheeled garment rack also can be useful, especially if your laundry room is on the same floor as your bedroom; you can push or pull the rack full of clothes instead of having to carry them.

If your laundry room is in the basement or if your bedroom and hamper are on a different floor and you don't have a laundry shoot, try tossing dirty clothes down the stairs instead of carrying them. You can use a grabber tool (more on that in the "Tools to help you move your stuff around" section, later in this chapter) to pick them up when you get downstairs. For carting laundry upstairs, consider using a wheeled grocery cart or laundry basket — or ask someone else in your household to bring it up.

Tools to help you get around

The weakness often associated with COPD can make even a short walk — say, from the living room to the bathroom — difficult and frightening. Canes and walkers can provide stability and support.

If you're using a walker, it's even more important that your pathways be wide and clear (see "Reorganizing things you use often," earlier in this chapter). Continually bumping into things is frustrating — and it can be dangerous if you lose your balance and fall.

Walkers with wheels generally are easier to move, because you don't have to pick them up with every step. However, some people feel less secure with these models, at least at first. If you prefer a walker without wheels, you can attach furniture coasters to the legs so you can slide it along the floor instead of picking it up with each step. Furniture coasters work well on carpeted floors because they slide along the surface, but they can be slippery on uncarpeted floors. If you don't have carpets, you can cut tennis balls in half and use them as coasters; they'll glide easily but still provide some traction, and they won't scuff your floor.

Motorized scooters, which are sold under a variety of names, are useful for moving around your home if you have large areas to cover and plenty of room to maneuver among your furnishings. They cost several thousand dollars, and not all insurance plans cover them. If you decide this option would be a good fit in your home, check with your doctor or insurer about your coverage. Your insurance company may require certification that you're unable to walk on your own.

Tools to help you move your stuff around

Medical supply stores sell baskets that attach to your walker, so you can move stuff from room to room without having to carry it yourself. Many retailers also sell collapsible grocery carts that you can push or drag behind you; these carts can be useful in the home for moving laundry or any number of other things.

Grabber tools allow you to reach things high and low without stretching or bending. They typically consist of a long handle and a trigger mechanism that opens and closes a grip device. Most of them are good for picking up things from the floor, pulling clothes out of the dryer, and doing other tasks around the house.

Use caution with grabber tools. Some are too flimsy to reliably hold anything with any heft to it, and you don't want to risk pulling a heavy crystal serving dish from the top shelf of your cabinet and having it crash to the floor or, worse, on you.

Simplify, Simplify

Sometimes people think they have to do things the hard way; otherwise, they tell themselves, it's not worthwhile. Remind yourself that it's okay to do things the easy way sometimes, especially when you have a good reason. And COPD is one of those good reasons. Your body uses so much more energy to breathe that any additional physical strain can cause real problems. Keeping things simple is an essential part of protecting your health.

Keeping meals simple

Preparing food can take a lot of energy, and COPD sufferers often find themselves too tired to eat after they've made their meals. You can make food preparation easier by planning ahead, using labor-saving appliances, and employing easy cleanup tricks.

Planning ahead

You can save time and energy by gathering all the materials you need to fix your meal before you start the work. With your ingredients, utensils, spices, and pans right in front of you, you eliminate the need to make several trips around the kitchen.

Schedule rest periods into your meal preparation schedule. You may want to take a break after you've gathered the fixings for your meal and before you start actually preparing it. You may want to take another break after preparing it before you start eating. And, because digestion takes a lot of energy that can make breathing more difficult, always plan to rest after eating.

By doubling or tripling recipes, you can cook once and get several meals out of your labor. Use freezer bags or individual containers to freeze leftovers; you'll have your own one-step microwave or boil-in-a-bag meals handy for those times when you just don't feel up to cooking.

Labor-saving appliances

Microwaves, toaster ovens, and crockpots or slow cookers are particularly useful when you have COPD because they are usually at counter height, they don't have to be tended the way stovetop pans do, and they don't heat up the kitchen the way ovens do. The exception to this is the over-the-stove microwave that doubles as a range hood and exhaust fan. If your kitchen is equipped with one of these and it's hard for you to reach, consider investing in a countertop model. You still can (and should) use the exhaust fan function on your existing microwave, but a countertop model will be easier for you to use for everyday cooking.

Easy cleanup tricks

Cleaning up after a meal sometimes is more work than making the meal. You can significantly reduce your labor by using aluminum foil to line baking pans and plastic liners for your crockpot; both virtually eliminate the need to scrub pots and pans. When items do need scrubbing, let them soak first in hot, soapy water to loosen the food as much as possible.

If you don't have a dishwasher, let dishes air-dry. If it's practical for you, reset the table with dry dishes instead of putting them in the cupboard; you eliminate two extra steps that way. Likewise, if you'll be using a pot or skillet again soon, keep it on the stove instead of stowing it in the cabinet.

If you do have a dishwasher, collect all the dishes that need to be washed before you begin loading; this eliminates unnecessary movement. Also, try sitting down while you load the washer. You won't have to bend as far, so breathing should be easier this way.

Quick cleaning tips

Dust is a pesky irritant at the best of times, and it's especially irritating when you have COPD. Unfortunately, the cleaning products that most people use for keeping dust under control pose their own problems for those with COPD: Feather dusters just kick the dust into the air, and the fumes from furniture polish and other cleaners can be just as irritating to the lungs as the dust itself, if not more so. That said, though, there are a few things you can use to keep your home neat without using up a lot of energy or making it harder for you to breathe.

Dusting

Feather dusting is out, and polish can irritate your lungs. So what are your options? You can try special dust cloths that grab the dust without the use of furniture polish; Pledge and Swiffer are two popular brands. If they don't do the job for you, consider wearing a mask while you dust with polish to reduce the amount of fumes you inhale. In fact, you may want to wear a mask whether you use polish or dry-dust; it doesn't hurt.

Carpet sweepers

Motorized or not, carpet sweepers are useful for quick cleanup of crumbs and dry spills. They weigh much less than a conventional vacuum so they're easier to push and pull, and they have long handles so you don't have to bend. Most of them also work on hard surfaces. One disadvantage: They don't work particularly well on exceptionally thick carpet or ones with long strands, like shag.

Mops and brooms

Dry mops and brooms generally are not recommended when you have COPD because they can swirl dust particles, pet hair, and other irritants into the air, making it harder to breathe. Sponge mops can retain moisture, making them susceptible to mildew — another dangerous irritant when you have COPD.

Your best bet is to invest in one of the new mops, such as the Swiffer WetJet or the Clorox ReadyMop, that uses disposable pads and a spray cleaning solution (get an unscented variety if possible). Although they may not satisfy the neat freak in you, they're good enough for small cleanups. They're also lightweight and easy to move along the floor, so using them doesn't take a lot of energy.

If you feel you have to use a broom, try fastening a damp cloth around it to collect dust and small particles. Get a dustpan with a long handle so you don't have to bend to sweep stuff into it; these are available at most major retailers.

Creating a social center

When it's time to visit with family and friends, you want a place that's comfortable and convenient, whether it's the kitchen table or the living room. Organize furniture so everyone can make eye contact easily; remove large centerpieces that obstruct face-to-face views, for instance, and place chairs at angles so people don't have to bend forward or twist themselves around to look at each other.

Keep your visiting area free of clutter to create a more welcoming atmosphere. Put large pillows and throw blankets beside the couch or along the back so people can sit down freely. Use baskets or lazy Susans to keep items on tables from scattering over the whole surface. Keep books and magazines stacked neatly, and winnow them periodically.

Do what you can to minimize background noise while you're visiting:

- Mute the TV.
- Turn fans and air conditioners on low.
- Keep your oxygen equipment in good working order so it doesn't groan or gurgle at your guests.

Finally, invite your guests to help themselves to beverages and snacks. It's easier for them to get up and get these things, and they won't mind. In fact, friends and family likely will object if you make any effort to wait on them, so you don't have to feel guilty about establishing a "self-serve" rule.

On the Level

Even a few steps can seem like Mount Everest when you can't catch your breath. Unfortunately, we live in a multilevel world, which means you may have to get creative about moving from one level to another.

Minimize trips up and down stairs

Planning ahead can save you a lot of exertion and stress, and nowhere is this more evident than when it comes to going up and down stairs. Frequent trips up to the bedroom or down to the basement can rob you of energy you need to breathe and can even trigger acute symptoms. Of course, avoiding these trips isn't always possible, but there are things you can do to make them less common.

Duplicate your supplies

Keep a set of commonly used supplies on each level of your home. For example, you should have a manicure set for upstairs and one for downstairs. The same applies to things like first-aid kits, pens and paper, perhaps even makeup and toiletries, depending on your routine. You can brush your teeth and comb your hair downstairs, for example, if you have an extra set of supplies in the downstairs bath.

You may want to keep an extra pair of slippers on the ground floor, so you don't have to go upstairs to change into them after returning from an outing. If you like to take an afternoon nap, keep a bed pillow and light blanket in the living room so you can nap on the couch if you don't feel like climbing the stairs.

Rearrange your routine

Changing the order in which you do things so you don't have to tackle the stairs so often may make sense. If you prefer to wash and dress after breakfast, for instance, can you do it in the downstairs bathroom? If you don't have a shower or tub downstairs, would it be easier for you to change your routine so you wash and dress before breakfast? Or maybe it would make sense for your schedule to shower at night instead. Experiment with your routine to figure out the alterations that work best for you.

Carry it with you

Getting duplicates of things like eyeglasses and medications can be expensive, and you probably don't want to keep one copy of the book you're reading upstairs and another copy downstairs. But you can get into the habit of carrying these things downstairs with you each day so you don't have to fetch them later; taking them back upstairs at night can become a part of your regular before-bed routine.

A large fanny pack may be all you need, depending on how much you want to carry with you. A fanny pack keeps your hands free, which is important if you worry about your balance on the stairs. You just have to make sure the belt isn't too tight.

Another option is a tote bag, like the ones people take to the beach. These hold quite a bit, and you can loop the handles over your forearm or let the bottom of the bag rest on the stairs and gently drag it behind you.

Install handy ramps

Ramps generally are easier to navigate than stairs, especially if you have moderate or severe COPD. Moving up or down the gentle slope of a properly installed ramp doesn't require as much energy, and it's much easier to pull oxygen tanks or wheeled carts along a ramp than up and down steps.

Because there are so many technical and regulatory issues involved in building a ramp, we don't recommend that you do it yourself. A professional will know local building codes, the best materials to use for the climate you live in, and how to make the ramp most useful for your needs.

However, even if you hire a professional, there are some things you should keep in mind. One is how you want the ramp to fit with other exterior features of your home. Do you already have a deck in place, for example? If not, do you want to add a larger landing area at the door that can double as a porch or deck? How wide do you want the ramp to be?

Figuring slope

Your builder likely will use some terms that may not be familiar to you. One is *slope* (the rate of incline from one end of the ramp to the other). The steeper the slope of a ramp, the more difficult it is to go up and down. The Americans with Disabilities Act (ADA) calls for a maximum slope of 1 inch of rise for every 12 inches of ramp. This is expressed as a ratio, 1:12, and it means that one end of your ramp goes up 1 inch vertically for every foot of its length (see Figure 14-1). One end of a 4-foot-long ramp, then, should only be 4 inches higher than the other end. If you want a gentler slope, you can use 1 inch of rise for every 18 inches of ramp (or a 1:18 ratio).

Figure 14-1:
The length
of your ramp
depends on
the height of
your door.

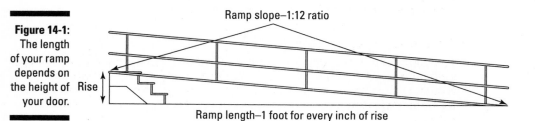

Ramp slope—1:12 ratio

Rise

Ramp length—1 foot for every inch of rise

Here's another way to express it: You need 12 inches of ramp for every 1 inch of height. So, if your door is 3½ feet off the ground, or 42 inches high, your ramp needs to be 504 feet long (42 × 12). Most properties don't have enough room to use a straight ramp that long, which is where turns and landing areas come in (making hiring a professional all that much more important).

Landing areas, handrails, and width

The ADA requires that *landing areas* (the platforms at the top and bottom of ramps) be at least 5 feet long. If the landing area is placed at a turn in the ramp, it must be at least 5 feet long by 5 feet wide; this is so wheelchairs have enough room to maneuver around the turn.

Handrails should be at least 32 inches above the ramp; this makes them easy for adults to use. The ADA also recommends that they be spaced 3 feet apart, so you can easily reach both of them. But a 3-foot-wide ramp may not suit your needs, particularly if you're using a wheelchair or a motorized scooter. Even if you don't need a wheelchair, it may make sense to install a wider ramp to accommodate your oxygen tank or wheeled grocery cart.

When you have to stretch and bend

Stretching and bending can be real chores when you have COPD. No matter how well you organize your home, you won't always be able to avoid stretching or bending. But you can pace your activities so you don't have to do a lot of either all at once.

Spread out your cleaning

Cleaning the closet or the pantry or the refrigerator is a day's task at the best of times. When you have COPD, though, it's better to break these kinds of jobs into much smaller chunks and spread them out over several days. When the fridge needs to be cleaned out, do one shelf or drawer today, another tomorrow, and so on until you've hit them all. The same goes for the closet: Clean the floor of the closet today, the middle shelves tomorrow, and the upper rack the day after. Breaking up bigger jobs keeps you from overexerting yourself, which can help you ward off acute attacks.

Avoid exertion after meals

The digestion process often makes breathing harder, so be sure to put off any strenuous activities until well after you've eaten. If you can, do jobs that require stretching and bending before meals, and be sure to schedule enough downtime between that activity and meal preparation so you don't tire yourself.

Practice new techniques

The way you stretch and bend can affect how it makes you feel. Instead of bending at the waist with both feet on the ground, try using the golfer's bend, in which you support yourself with your left hand on a wall, counter, or chair, and bend with your right leg straight behind you, using your right hand to reach (see Figure 14-2). If you're left-handed, support yourself with your right hand and stretch your left leg out behind you. Using opposite limbs (right hand/left leg or left hand/right leg) helps with balance.

The golfer's bend is not a good technique if you have trouble balancing. If you feel like you may fall, or if it just isn't comfortable for you, don't use this method.

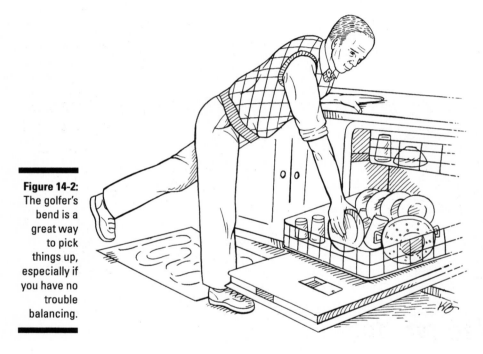

Figure 14-2:
The golfer's bend is a great way to pick things up, especially if you have no trouble balancing.

Another way to get to ground level without bending at the waist is to crouch your way down. Follow these steps (shown in Figure 14-3):

1. **Place your feet a little more than shoulder-width apart.**

2. **Bend your knees until you're in a crouching position, on the balls of your feet.**

3. **If you still can't reach what you want, drop to one or both knees.**

4. **Rise to a standing position, keeping your back straight.**

The advantage of this technique is that it keeps your back straight, so it doesn't interfere with breathing the way bending over can.

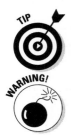

Use this technique when you have something to hold onto — a counter or solid piece of furniture. This will help you keep your balance.

If you suffer from arthritis or other joint pain, the crouching bend may not work for you. The golfer's bend, described earlier in this section, may be a better option.

Figure 14-3:
Crouching is another great way to pick up things on the floor without interfering with your breathing.

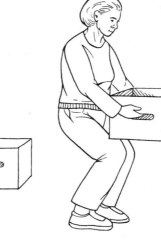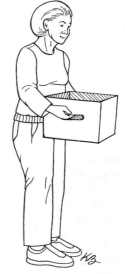

Asking for Help

Sometimes you just don't have the energy or inclination to do the things you used to do. Admitting that you need help is difficult. Sometimes admitting that you *want* help is even harder. Asking for help may make you feel discouraged, worthless, or like you're a burden to others.

Remember two things: Everyone needs a hand now and then, so you're just proving your humanity when you need assistance. And people like to help others; they get a lift from doing good for the ones they love, especially when they feel as though their help was wanted.

Calling on family and friends

Relatives and friends often feel powerless and frustrated because they can't fix the problem or make the COPD patient feel better. You can help ease those feelings by asking them to do things that are specific, constructive, and helpful.

A family member who lives with you may take over responsibility for meal planning or cooking. One who doesn't live with you may take you out grocery shopping once a week and help you put the groceries away when you get home.

You can ask friends to take you to appointments at the hairdresser's or doctor's office. They may even be willing to come over and help you pack away your winter wardrobe and get out your summer clothes. Maybe they can put out the trash for you or do similar quick chores that are beyond your strength.

Outsourcing chores

Some regular chores are too demanding to expect your loved ones to do all the time. After all, you don't want them to resent the time or energy they spend helping you. For things like lawn care, snow shoveling, house painting, and other jobs, hiring someone to do it for you on a regular basis may be a better option.

You may want to hire a maid service to do regular cleaning so you don't have to deal with the exertion or the cleaning products. Many services will do the whole gamut or will customize their service to your needs. If you can handle the dusting and vacuuming, for example, you may want to hire someone to come in weekly or every other week to clean the bathrooms and kitchen. You can also hire these firms (or individuals) to do one-time projects like spring cleaning.

If you can't afford to pay someone to do these things for you, check with your church or local volunteer agencies. Government social service agencies may also be able to refer you to free or low-cost services.

When it's time for a home aide

When you regularly have difficulty doing routine daily tasks — not just a bad day here and there, but strings of bad days and fewer and fewer good days — it's time to consider bringing in daily help. Depending on your needs, you may be able to use a personal or home aide. If you need help with medications and the like, you probably need a home health aide.

Both personal aides and home health aides usually work under the supervision of a registered nurse. Their goal is to help you continue living in your home, rather than in a nursing home or other healthcare facility, even if you need daily help to stay in your home.

Personal or home aides generally provide help with housekeeping and daily living tasks. They may help you bathe and get dressed, for instance, if you have difficulty doing it on your own. They may grocery-shop for you or prepare meals in advance. They may run errands or take you to and from appointments. They'll also do laundry, change the bed, straighten the house, and so on.

Home health aides perform more health-related functions than housekeeping services. They administer medicines, check your vital signs, and help you do your exercises. They also help you move from one room or chair to another, and they may do some light picking up around the house.

Your doctor can refer you to agencies that provide home care services, or you can look in your phone book under "Home Health Care." Many agencies offer free in-home consultations to determine how often an aide would visit you, what he would do, and how much it would cost. Some insurance plans pay for these services, too.

Check the licensing requirements for home health aides in your state, and make sure the agency you hire and its employees are properly qualified to deliver the care they promise. Most insurance plans will only pay for services from a qualified agency. Your doctor's office can help you find this information.

Chapter 15

Clearing the Air at Home

• •

• •

*W*hen you hear the words *air pollution,* you probably think of the thick yellow haze that sometimes hovers over large cities or the old factory stacks that belch thick columns of black smoke into the sky. In fact, the quality of the air you breathe indoors can be just as poor as the air quality outdoors; in some cases, indoor air is even worse. One recent study found that the pollution from improperly vented cooking stoves or fireplaces leads to as many as 1.5 million deaths worldwide every year. Granted, the vast majority of those deaths occur in poor and developing countries, but the rest of the world is by no means immune.

Most homes have more than one source of pollution, and, in many cases, it's the combination of pollutants, coupled with long-running exposure, that leads to problems. Irritants can make your eyes water, your nose run, and your throat sore. They can make you cough or sneeze. They can give you a headache or make you feel tired or dizzy. Over years, they can even cause or contribute to a range of health problems, including heart disease, cancer, and, yes, COPD. The problem is that, by the time you really sit up and take notice of your symptoms, the damage to your health may already be done.

COPD can make you more sensitive to air quality, no matter where you are. And, when you have COPD, the quality of the air around you is a crucial component of your overall sense of well-being. Poor indoor air can make you feel like it's even harder to catch your breath and may lead to sudden attacks. Those sudden attacks certainly will make you feel worse, even if they don't land you in the hospital, and there is some evidence to suggest that COPD patients with more frequent sudden attacks fare worse overall than those who have fewer attacks.

In this chapter, we identify some common household pollutants, from the familiar — dust mites, cleansers, and pesticides — to some that may surprise you, like the fumes your furniture may give off. We also provide some strategies for minimizing the irritants in your home's air and tell you which work best and which are, in most cases, a waste of time and money.

Types of Indoor Air Pollution

The air in your home can be chock-full of irritants from a number of sources. Most people think of their heating and cooling systems first; after all, dirty ducts can kick a whole lot of dust into the air around your favorite easy chair, and that's pollution you can see. But there are lots of sources you can't see. Or smell. Or taste.

In broad terms, indoor air pollution can come from biological sources, like mold, mildew, dust mites, pets, and pests; from gases, like carbon monoxide and radon; from chemicals in the cleaning supplies you use around the house and even your furnishings; and from combustion — that is, heating, cooling, and cooking, which can load the air with tiny particles of wood, oil, coal, or what have you.

Biological sources

Plants, pets, and people can fill the air in your home with all kinds of airborne irritants. Plants can release pollen, and the soil they're in can carry bacteria. Pet dander and saliva can trigger allergic reactions. When dry, urine and feces from pets and unwanted animals like mice and rats can become airborne. And, of course, people can transmit viruses and bacteria to each other.

Mold and mildew also are potent sources of indoor air pollution, which is one reason it's important to seal leaks in ceilings and around plumbing as soon as possible. Warmth and moisture provide ideal growing conditions for lots of bacteria, mildew, and insects, including dust mites. You can minimize these things by keeping the relative humidity in your home at between 30 percent and 60 percent.

Check your local hardware, department, or home improvement store for a *hygrometer* (a device that measures the relative humidity in your home). Many of the newer electronic room thermometers — and some mechanical devices — include relative humidity readings with the temperature reading. Cost can range from as little as $20 to $100 or more, depending on how fancy you want to get.

Common symptoms of biological indoor air pollution include coughing, watery eyes, and sneezing. Depending on how sensitive you are to these things, you also may experience shortness of breath, fever, dizziness, or even digestive problems.

Heating and cooling systems can become contaminated with biological irritants and cause something called *humidifier fever,* marked by a sudden fever and sometimes accompanied by achy muscles and shortness of breath. Although humidifier fever is most often associated with large buildings, it can occur at home if the heating or cooling system is contaminated with bacteria, fungi, or other organisms.

If your home tends to be damp, a dehumidifier might be a worthwhile investment. Just be sure to keep the water pan clean; bacteria and insects love standing water.

Gases

Your home may be full of noxious gases that can make breathing more difficult. Some, like carbon monoxide, you may be familiar with; others, like the fumes given off by dry cleaning and even the materials your furniture is made of, may surprise you.

Carbon monoxide

Carbon monoxide is probably the best-known indoor air threat, thanks in part to the proliferation of home carbon monoxide detectors. These are similar to home smoke detectors, except they monitor levels of the odorless, tasteless gas and alert you when those levels reach the danger zone. A carbon monoxide detector is an important complement to your smoke detector, because fires can give off potentially lethal levels of the gas before your smoke detector goes off.

But fires are far from the only source of carbon monoxide in your home. The most common household sources are unvented kerosene or propane space heaters, improperly maintained chimneys, furnaces, and gas stoves, and gas-powered generators or other gas-powered equipment.

Never idle your car or any other gas-powered vehicle or equipment in a closed garage. Remember, too, that carbon monoxide can seep into your home if your garage is attached to your house.

Carbon monoxide inhibits your ability to take in oxygen. A little carbon monoxide in the air you breathe may make you feel sleepy or cause chest pain, especially if you have heart disease. Low-level carbon monoxide poisoning often causes flu-like symptoms: headaches or muscle aches, nausea, confusion, and fatigue. At moderate levels, your vision may get blurry and you may feel disoriented or like you're going to pass out. High concentrations of carbon monoxide can be fatal.

Volatile organic compounds

Volatile organic compounds (VOCs) are emitted as gases from literally thousands of common household products: paint and varnish, paint strippers, cleaning solutions, glues, markers, office equipment, building materials, furnishings, and even cosmetics. Because VOCs are so common in the various things that we live and work around, concentrations are typically higher in the air indoors than out. An Environmental Protection Agency (EPA) study found that VOC levels were two to five times higher inside homes than outside, and the higher indoor concentration was found in both urban and rural homes.

VOCs can irritate your eyes, nose, and throat and can cause headaches or nausea. Other possible health effects include dizziness, fatigue, difficulty breathing, and, with long-term exposure, damage to your kidneys, liver, or central nervous system.

Nitrogen dioxide

Like carbon monoxide, nitrogen dioxide can get into your home through improperly installed or poorly maintained appliances like gas stoves and propane or kerosene space heaters. In homes with these appliances, indoor concentrations of nitrogen dioxide often are higher than outdoor air concentrations. If you don't have any of these appliances, the air in your home probably has about half the nitrogen dioxide levels of outdoor air. Nitrogen dioxide also is a common element in tobacco smoke and welding fumes.

Low-level exposure to nitrogen dioxide can irritate the linings in your eyes, nose, throat, and airways. If you have asthma in addition to COPD, you may be quite sensitive to nitrogen dioxide. Prolonged exposure can contribute to chronic bronchitis, or, if you already have COPD, decrease your lung function. Exposure to extremely high levels is rare, except in a building fire, but in those cases it can cause swelling and damage in the lungs.

Radon

Radon is another tasteless, odorless, colorless gas that can invade your home; it's a natural radioactive gas that is the leading cause of lung cancer in nonsmokers and the second-leading cause of lung cancer overall. Cancer caused by radon exposure claims some 20,000 lives a year in the United States.

Fireplaces, wood stoves, and kerosene heaters are the main culprits in high household radon levels. Radon exposure can irritate your eyes, nose, and throat. You may be more susceptible to respiratory infections and bouts of bronchitis. If you already have COPD, radon exposure will make it harder to breathe and may contribute to more frequent attacks of worse COPD symptoms.

Chemicals

You're probably familiar with the warnings on a variety of household chemicals that caution you to use them only in well-ventilated areas. Those warnings are on everything from bleach and floor cleaners to paint cans and bug sprays, because all of them can cause problems if you inhale high concentrations of their fumes.

Methylene chloride

Methylene chloride is a common chemical in paint strippers, aerosol spray paint, and products that remove glue and other adhesives. When you inhale methylene chloride, your body converts it into carbon monoxide, the same potentially lethal gas that comes out of your car exhaust. Symptoms of exposure to methylene chloride are similar to the symptoms of carbon monoxide exposure: fatigue, headache, dizziness, confusion, and, with prolonged exposure, blurred vision and loss of consciousness.

Benzene

Benzene is found in tobacco smoke, including second-hand smoke, as well as stored fuels (think of that five-gallon container of gas you keep in the garage for the lawn mower) and painting supplies. Benzene is known to cause cancer in humans, so it's a good idea to minimize your exposure to this chemical:

- ✔ Don't allow people to smoke in your home.
- ✔ Don't mix fuel for lawn mowers, weed cutters, or other items in enclosed spaces.
- ✔ Don't use painting supplies in unventilated areas.

Perchloroethylene

Perchloroethylene is commonly used in dry cleaning. As a rule, dry cleaners try to recapture as much of this chemical as they can during the cleaning process so they can use it again on the next batch of garments. But sometimes dry cleaners don't take as much perchloroethylene out of fabrics as they can. That means your clothing — or curtains or upholstery — gives off fumes from this chemical into the air around you, so you inhale it. If your dry cleaning has a strong chemical odor when you pick it up, it probably hasn't been dried properly. Your best bet is to insist on proper drying, or, if this happens often, to change dry cleaners.

Pesticides

Three-quarters of Americans use at least one pesticide in their homes at least once a year. Insecticides and disinfectants are potent poisons, used to get rid of bugs, termites, rodents, fungi, bacteria, and viruses. These chemicals don't get into your air only when you use them, though; they can contaminate the air when you store them, when they evaporate from the surfaces you use them on, or when they float or are tracked in from outdoor sources, like soil that has been treated with a pesticide. Some studies of home indoor air have found measurable levels of as many as 12 different pesticides.

The "active ingredient" listed on any given pesticide is not the only chemical that gets into your air. It's carried by any number of other ingredients, which aren't toxic to the pest you're trying to kill but which can have adverse affects on you. They may irritate your eyes, nose, and throat; cause coughing, nausea, headaches, or dizziness; even, with long-term exposure, harm your kidneys, liver, or central nervous system.

Mothballs contain a potent pesticide than can cause health problems in humans if the vapors are inhaled. That's why you should only use mothballs and other moth repellants in containers that can be stored well away from the occupied areas of your home: in a ventilated attic, for example, or a detached garage.

Formaldehyde

Most people associate formaldehyde with the funeral industry — it's used as part of the embalming process — but it also is widely used in construction and furniture manufacturing, and can be found in tobacco smoke, fuel-burning appliances, and some household products like adhesives and varnishes. Formaldehyde also is used in permanent-press clothing, linens, and drapes.

Two kinds of formaldehyde are used in construction and the making of furniture. *Urea-formaldehyde* resins — which, unfortunately, are more common in indoor furnishings and building materials — emit more formaldehyde into the air than *phenol-formaldehyde,* which is commonly used in exterior building materials.

Potential sources of formaldehyde in your home include

- ✔ Particleboard, commonly used in some-assembly-required furniture and as subflooring and shelving
- ✔ Hardwood paneling, either as wallcovering or in furniture

- ✔ Fiberboard, particularly the medium-density kind that's commonly used in furniture
- ✔ Permanent-press textiles
- ✔ Urea-formaldehyde foam insulation

Formaldehyde has a strong, pungent odor; if you ever dissected a frog in biology class, you'll recognize the smell. If not, think of the smell of brand-new carpet or a vinegary adhesive. Many people can detect formaldehyde's odor at very low levels, but some people don't smell it even at high levels. Symptoms of formaldehyde exposure include watery eyes or a burning sensation in the eyes, nose, or throat. At higher levels, exposure can cause headache, nausea, fatigue, and difficulty breathing; it can even trigger asthma attacks.

 Formaldehyde lingers in products long after they're manufactured, so even your older furnishings can give off formaldehyde vapors. More formaldehyde is emitted when temperatures and humidity are high, so you may find the vapors more troublesome in hot weather.

Particles

Any appliance that uses combustible fuel — wood, propane, kerosene, fuel oil — can release tiny particles into the air that you, in turn, can inhale. That's why it's so important to keep your furnace, wood stove, gas oven, gas-powered space heater, and other fuel-burning appliances in good working order. Furnaces should have maintenance checks every year to make sure they're adequately vented and that chimneys and flues are working properly.

 Tobacco smoke releases particles into the air, too. In fact, people who are around smokers may inhale more of these particles than the smokers themselves, because secondhand smoke isn't filtered.

When you breathe in particles from incompletely burned fuels, they can lodge in your lungs, irritating your airways and possibly damaging your lung tissue. In addition, pollutants like radon and benzene can attach themselves to these particles and take a ride inside your lungs.

At low levels or in brief, infrequent bursts, exposure to airborne particles can cause irritation in your eyes, nose, and throat. More prolonged exposure can contribute to respiratory infections and bronchitis. Depending on which chemicals attach themselves to the particles and how long you're exposed to them, breathing them in also can contribute to the development of lung cancer.

Cleaning the Air

Ridding your home of air pollution may sound like a daunting task, but in most cases it's relatively simple. There are three main strategies: eliminating the source of the pollution; improving ventilation in your home; and using air filters, air fresheners, and air purifiers. A combination of these methods will take care of most indoor household air-quality problems.

Eliminating the source

Getting rid of the thing that's emitting noxious vapors into your air isn't always possible. But, when it *is* possible, eliminating the source is the quickest and (usually) least expensive strategy to pursue.

Here are some ways you can minimize sources of pollution in your home:

- ✔ **Buy only what you can use.** Don't keep large amounts of painting supplies, pesticides, adhesives, or cleaners around; fumes can leak out of even closed containers.

- ✔ **Throw away what you don't need.** Regularly clean out cans of old paint, paint thinners, sealants, adhesives, and the like.

- ✔ **Store items away from living areas.** If you have leftover paint, pesticides, or what have you, store the containers in a cool, dry place away from where you spend most of your time. Ventilated attics or garages are ideal; unventilated areas are the least desirable.

- ✔ **Have your heating and cooling systems checked regularly.** Improperly working furnaces, air conditioners, fireplaces, and wood stoves can increase the levels of various gases and particles in your indoor air. Wet coils on cooling systems can promote the growth of mold. Have a certified technician check these things every year to make sure they're clean and working properly.

    Regular maintenance of your heating and cooling systems will extend the life of those systems and improve their efficiency, as well as eliminate potential sources of air pollution.

- ✔ **Make sure gas appliances are properly adjusted.** Improperly adjusted gas stoves emit more carbon monoxide and other gases than ones that are properly adjusted. Gas jets should be checked regularly to make sure they aren't clogged.

Improving ventilation

Indoor pollutants can build up relatively easily if you don't get enough air from outdoors into your home. In fact, when it comes to indoor air quality, an "airtight" house is less desirable than a "leaky" house. But even leaky houses can have poor indoor air quality when weather conditions prevent air from moving in and out.

According to the EPA, there are some telltale signs that your home doesn't have adequate ventilation:

✔ Condensation on windows or walls

✔ Stuffy, stale, or smelly air

✔ Areas where books, shoes, or other items are prone to develop mold

✔ Dirty heating and cooling systems

There are three ways to get outdoor air inside: infiltration, natural ventilation, and mechanical ventilation. The first two are the easiest and least expensive; the last, though it can be expensive, is especially good in homes that are damp because it can help prevent growth of mold and mildew.

Heat and humidity are the prime ingredients for developing mold and attracting many kinds of insects. Keeping the humidity level below 50 percent in attics, cellars, and crawl spaces can prevent moisture from building up in your walls, ceilings, floors, and insulation.

Infiltration

Outdoor air can get into your home through the joins of floors and walls or windows and doors, and through cracks and tiny openings in walls and roofs. This process is called *infiltration;* air can sneak in from the outside even if you don't feel any drafts. Most people think air infiltration is a bad thing, mainly because your heating and cooling systems may use more energy and work harder to keep the air inside at a comfortable temperature. But the addition of outdoor air can help dilute the concentrations of indoor air pollutants, making them less irritating to you. So resist the urge to seal up your home as if it were a hazardous waste site. A little infiltration is a good thing.

Natural ventilation

This is just a fancy term for opening the doors and windows in your home. Airing out your house this way can get rid of a lot of pollutants, or at least lower their concentrations to levels where they won't bother you. It also can help get rid of odors from cooking, burning fuel (as in a fireplace or wood stove), and other sources.

The movement of air through infiltration and natural ventilation depends on wind and on differences in the temperature between the air outdoors and the air inside. If there's no wind and the temperatures indoors and out are more or less the same, there will be little exchange of air. A breeze and a temperature difference of at least a few degrees creates a better exchange of outdoor and indoor air.

Mechanical ventilation

You probably have some mechanical ventilation built into your home: an exhaust fan in the bathroom, for instance, and one over the stove in the kitchen. These systems, when they are vented to your home's exterior, are pretty good at removing air from the room they serve and bringing outdoor air into the room. Vents on window air conditioners and attic fans — sometimes called house fans or whole-house fans — perform a similar function, drawing indoor air out and outdoor air in.

Some newer central heating and cooling systems also are designed to bring outside air in, but, unless you live in a new house, chances are your furnace and air conditioning system don't do this. Even forced-air systems don't exchange indoor and outdoor air; they just recycle the indoor air.

Kitchen and bathroom exhaust fans are designed to remove pollutants, odors, and moisture from the air. When they're used regularly, they can help keep your indoor air cleaner.

Ventilation is particularly important when you're using products that produce a lot of fumes, like paint, paint thinner or stripper, varnishes, and glue. If possible, use these things only near an open door or window; if you have to use them in an enclosed space, use a fan to keep the air circulating.

Using fresheners, filters, and purifiers

Thousands of products claim to freshen, filter, and purify the air in your home. Air fresheners alone — in the form of sprays, solids, plug-ins, scented candles, and oils — are a $1.7 billion business in the United States. Then there are any number of filters and so-called air purifiers that run the gamut in both price and effectiveness.

When you have COPD, keeping the air inside your home as clean as possible is important. But it's also important to weigh the pros and cons of the products aimed at keeping your home's air fresh and clean. Some products just aren't worth the money or the time you'll spend using them. And some can be downright harmful to you.

Air fresheners

About three-quarters of American households use some kind of air freshener regularly. But not all air fresheners are created equal. Many of them contain chemicals called *phthalates,* which may cause cancer at high exposure levels. In fact, some phthalates have been banned in more than a dozen countries (but not yet in the United States). Phthalates aren't regulated by the Food and Drug Administration and do not have to be included on labels, so there's no easy way to know whether the product you're using contains them.

Another problem for COPD sufferers is the fragrances themselves. You may find yourself becoming more sensitive to strongly scented sprays and candles; if you have asthma in addition to COPD, your sensitivity may be even higher, and exposure to certain air fresheners may trigger an asthmatic attack. In other cases, you may get a headache or have trouble breathing when air fresheners are used.

You can keep odors under control without emptying your wallet. Sprinkle baking soda in the bottom of trash cans, especially in the kitchen. Keep a small bowl of ground coffee on the kitchen counter. If drain odors are a problem, try grinding up half a lemon in your garbage disposal, or pour a tablespoon or two of coffee grounds (after you've brewed the coffee) into the drain and wash them down with hot tap water.

If you decide to use air fresheners, stick with unscented or lightly scented sprays, and don't use them too frequently. Turn on exhaust fans when using sprays in kitchens and bathrooms.

Air filters

Air filters come in all qualities and price ranges. In recent years, HEPA filters have grown enormously in popularity, especially among people with asthma or allergies. HEPA filters also can be useful for people with COPD, because they trap smaller airborne particles that can irritate your lungs.

HEPA stands for *high-efficiency particulate air.* A HEPA filter is designed to trap virtually all tiny airborne particles, including pollen and dust-mite feces. Such filters are available for furnaces, air conditioners, vacuums, and other appliances. They generally are more expensive than traditional paper filters, but they also are more effective at trapping both large and small particles.

To be effective in vacuums, all air has to be directed through the HEPA filter; otherwise, the particles get kicked back into the air just as they do with regular vacuums. Because HEPA filters are so much more dense than regular filters, HEPA vacuums have to have a more powerful motor to force air through the filter.

HEPA filters in furnaces and air conditioners also may become clogged more quickly than regular filters because they collect more airborne particles.

Check the filters on your furnace and air conditioner once a month, even if they're labeled for longer use. If a filter is dirty, change it; dirty filters restrict air flow and force your heating and cooling systems to work harder and less efficiently.

Air purifiers

Air purifying machines are not recommended for COPD patients because nearly all of them produce some amount of ozone, which is extremely harmful to your lungs. Even ionizers, which use electrically charged ions to collect and trap airborne particles, produce some ozone. Even though the amounts are tiny, it's not worth the risk when you have COPD.

Chapter 16

Preparing for Emergencies

. . . .

. . . .

*Y*our doctor calls the sudden onset of severe COPD symptoms an *acute exacerbation,* but hardly anyone outside the medical community uses that term. In fact, one study showed that fewer than 2 percent of patients understand what an exacerbation is; patients typically describe such an episode as a "crisis" — a much more sensible term, conveying as it does the suggestion of a scary emergency requiring immediate action.

That's the essence of suddenly severe symptoms. These attacks aren't harmless; they're extraordinarily frightening, and they have serious consequences for your immediate health and your long-term well-being. COPD flare-ups nearly always require additional medication and often result in hospitalization. It can take weeks or even months to fully recover from a sudden attack, and, unfortunately, some people never do regain their earlier health. The more often you have these attacks, the faster your health declines and the longer it takes you to recover from each episode.

Immediate and appropriate treatment can lessen the danger and perhaps even the long-range effects of COPD flare-ups. Unfortunately, some people ignore worsening symptoms until they reach the crisis stage, and that makes treatment and recovery more difficult. If you know what to watch out for and what to do when warning signs appear, you increase your chances of getting through a COPD crisis in relatively good condition.

In this chapter, we define the symptoms and common causes of sudden COPD attacks, and we walk you through some of the treatments you may receive if you have an attack. We show you how to create an action plan so you're well-prepared in the event of an emergency. And we give you some tips on preventing sudden attacks.

Suddenly Severe Symptoms

An acute exacerbation is a sudden worsening of your COPD symptoms. Your airways contract in a process doctors call *bronchospasm,* usually accompanied by swelling and increased mucus production. You may start coughing more violently and coughing up more mucus, and your mucus may change color, which can indicate infection. If you don't usually have wheezing, you may suddenly notice it; if you usually do have some wheezing, you may notice it's worse. The same is true for feeling short of breath; you may be aware of it for the first time during a sudden attack, or, if you've had some shortness of breath all along, it will be worse during a sudden attack.

Although COPD crises come on suddenly, they don't get resolved nearly as quickly. Worsened symptoms can last a few days to several weeks, and the toll they take on your overall health can last even longer.

COPD isn't easily predicted, and neither are sudden flare-ups. Some patients with severe COPD may not have frequent attacks or even any attacks at all, while some people with less severe COPD may have such attacks routinely. Many COPD patients start out experiencing one or two of these attacks a year. But as you age and as your COPD progresses, you can expect sudden attacks to get more frequent and, very likely, more severe.

Defining a crisis

The generally accepted medical definition of an acute exacerbation is "a sustained worsening of the patient's condition, from the stable state and beyond normal day-to-day variations, that is acute in onset and necessitates a change in regular medication in a patient with underlying COPD."

Interestingly, the definition itself points out the difficulty of coming up with universal guidelines for defining a sudden attack: Everyone with COPD has symptoms that can vary from one day to the next or even from one part of the day to the next, and everyone has his own concept of what constitutes "worse."

Add to that mix the fact that sudden attacks may be mild, moderate, or severe, and you can see why it's impossible to say, "You are having a COPD crisis when you experience *x, y,* and *z.*"

We can, however, offer some guidelines to help you assess the severity of your sudden attacks. These degrees of severity are defined by how the attack is treated:

- ✔ **Mild attacks** involve only one of the three main symptoms of a sudden attack (coughing up more mucus, changes in mucus that indicate infection, or intensified feelings of being short of breath) and at least one of the following conditions: increased wheezing or coughing, elevated heart or breathing rate, fever with no known cause, or a recent upper-respiratory infection. Mild attacks usually can be managed at home.

- ✔ **Moderate attacks** have at least two of the three main symptoms and require additional medications to treat; for these attacks, you'll probably call your doctor but won't feel the need to call an ambulance.

- ✔ **Severe attacks** have all three main symptoms and make you feel as though your health is rapidly declining. These attacks require immediate medical attention (ambulance or emergency room) and almost always result in a hospital stay.

What causes them

The most common cause of sudden COPD flare-up is infection, but other things can trigger attacks, too. Allergens like pollen, mold, and pet dander can make your symptoms suddenly worse; so can pollutants like tobacco smoke and ozone, and exposure to chemical fumes like paint thinner and varnish.

About half of acute COPD attacks are caused by bacteria or viruses that cause flu and pneumonia.

Infections may be the most common cause of sudden attacks for two reasons. First, COPD suppresses your immune system, so you're more vulnerable to airborne viruses and bacteria. Second, the extra mucus that your COPD produces is an excellent breeding ground for viruses and bacteria.

Green or yellow mucus doesn't always indicate an infection, but if you also have other symptoms like a fever, increased coughing, or feeling like it's harder to catch your breath, you should call your doctor.

Other complications

Aside from respiratory infections, COPD can cause other complications that should be evaluated by your doctor as quickly as possible:

- ✔ **Heart and circulatory complications:** COPD can cause a specific type of heart failure called *cor pulmonale,* or right heart failure. Cor pulmonale raises the risk of blood clots, because blood tends to pool in the right ventricle and in the legs. Watch for swelling in your feet, ankles, and legs.

- ✔ **Collapsed lung:** The medical term for this is *pneumothorax.* In COPD, it occurs when lung tissue is so damaged that a hole develops, allowing air to escape from the lung into your chest cavity and collapsing the lung. Symptoms include sharp chest pain (often only on the affected side), sudden difficulty breathing, pain when you breathe, tightness in your chest, and a rapid heartbeat. This can be life-threatening if not addressed quickly. If it isn't treated thoroughly, it can limit your ability to travel by plane or even visit places at high altitudes.

- ✔ **Too many red blood cells:** This condition, called *secondary polycythemia,* is unusual, but it does occur occasionally in COPD patients. Essentially, the deficiency of oxygen in your blood can prompt your body to create more red blood cells than it needs in an effort to distribute more oxygen. Symptoms include vision problems, such as distortion, blind spots, or flashes of light; bleeding in the gums or from minor cuts; and burning sensations in your hands or feet.

Preventing Sudden Attacks

Given the potentially serious consequences of COPD flare-ups, your best strategy is to try to prevent them from occurring in the first place. Of course, you can't always control the things that may spark a sudden worsening of your symptoms, but you can at least minimize your risk.

What you can do

The most effective prevention technique is taking care of yourself. That means you need to:

- ✔ **Quit smoking and avoid secondhand smoke.** The longer you smoke, the more damage you do to your lungs, and the more damaged your lungs are, the greater your chances of experiencing sudden breathing crises. (See Chapter 10 for information on how smoking affects your lungs and various methods of quitting.) Secondhand smoke is just as dangerous, even if you've already quit smoking yourself, so make your home a smoke-free zone and avoid smoky places like bars.

- ✔ **Pay attention to the air quality around you.** Stay indoors on days when there are ozone warnings or smog or other air pollution is high. The same goes for windy days when pollen and dust levels may be high. Hot, humid weather can make breathing more difficult, and so can very cold air temperatures.

✔ **Take advantage of flu shots and pneumonia vaccines.** Unless you have certain allergies, you should get a yearly flu shot and a pneumonia vaccination once every five years. (Ask your doctor if these pose any risk for you.)

✔ **Avoid people who have colds, coughs, or flu.** If you can't avoid them altogether — if a member of your household is ill or if a bug is making the rounds at your workplace, for instance — take precautions to protect yourself from catching what they've got. Don't share glasses or utensils; wash your hands frequently; use a hand sanitizer when you can't wash your hands.

✔ **Stick with your wellness program.** Eating right, getting plenty of rest, and exercising not only help control your daily COPD symptoms, they're especially important in helping your body defend itself against infection.

✔ **Keep your body hydrated.** Unless your doctor restricts your fluid intake, drinking plenty of water is a good way to keep mucus thin and easier to cough up. Maintaining a comfortable level of humidity in your home can help reduce chest congestion, too.

Why it matters

Acute exacerbations can be life-threatening. Up to 15 percent of patients with advanced COPD die in hospitals every year as a result of a severe attack, and up to 40 percent of them die within a year after suffering a severe attack.

The reasons for this aren't clearly understood, but suddenly severe symptoms seem to speed up the progression of COPD in many people. In other words, a sudden attack apparently causes even more damage to your lungs and the rest of your body, so every time you have one, you end up at least a little worse off than you were before the attack. The effects of any sudden attack last a long time, and the damage they do to your general health may not be fully reversible.

One theory is that these attacks cause structural damage to the lungs, which, in turn, speeds up the progression of COPD. Studies have shown, though, that while lung function improves within a few weeks after an attack is properly treated, other measures of overall health can take six months or more to improve. More-frequent attacks — more than two a year — generally result in faster declines of overall health.

Whatever the reason, over time, treatments for sudden attacks become less effective, and recovery becomes more problematic.

There's also the financial cost involved. More than half of the direct costs of COPD come from hospital admissions for treatment of sudden attacks. Hospitalization and more medications means higher co-pays for you — not to mention the anxiety and stress they cause for you and your loved ones.

Treating Sudden Attacks

As we note earlier in this chapter (see "Defining a crisis"), treatment of your COPD flare-ups will depend on their severity and, in many cases, what triggered the attack. Mild attacks generally can be treated at home. Moderate attacks may require a visit to the doctor, perhaps some tests and additional, short-term medications. Severe attacks require immediate medical attention and usually involve a hospital stay of at least a day or two.

Sometimes the toughest part of treating a sudden flare-up is identifying what caused it. You can do your part by telling your doctor about any circumstances that may have led to your symptoms getting worse — if you were exposed to secondhand smoke, for example, or in contact with someone who had a cold or other illness. A clear description of your symptoms can help your doctor clear up the mystery, too.

Your doctor may order tests like a sputum (mucus) culture or a chest X-ray to confirm the diagnosis or rule out certain possibilities. But, in many cases, you'll start treatment for your attack before the results of such tests are available.

At home

Mild and even moderate attacks usually don't require emergency medical care or hospitalization. Instead, your doctor may change the dose of medications you're already taking, substitute a new drug, or add short-term or maintenance medications to your treatment program.

If an attack is caused by a bacterial infection, your doctor will prescribe antibiotics; in fact, because it can be difficult to tell whether a respiratory infection is caused by bacteria or a virus, your doctor may give you antibiotics in any case. She may want you to take them for at least a few days as a preventive measure even if you don't have an infection. She also may recommend a short course of oral steroids to help you recover from the effects of your attack.

Finally, your doctor may recommend oxygen therapy (usually to help treat a serious attack that required hospitalization) or increase the flow rate or hours per day if you're already using oxygen. (See Chapter 8 for detailed information about various COPD medicines and oxygen therapy.)

In the ambulance, emergency room, or hospital

When your attacks are severe enough to warrant emergency medical care, your course of treatment will follow a general protocol. In an ambulance or emergency room, you'll be given bronchodilators to open your airways, steroids (in either oral or IV form) to reduce swelling, antibiotics if you've got a bacterial infection, and oxygen.

In emergency situations, oxygen can be administered through simple nasal cannulas or full masks — the kind you often see on TV medical shows. Both of these assist only in increasing the amount of oxygen you get. A more extreme option is *intubation,* a procedure in which a tube is placed in the windpipe to help the patient with the *gas exchange* (expelling carbon dioxide and taking in oxygen), which, in turn, helps reduce the work of breathing. Laypeople often refer to intubation as "life support."

Noninvasive ventilation

An oxygen mask is a noninvasive form of mechanical ventilation. The mask forms a seal around your mouth and nose (or, in some cases, around the nose only) and you inhale and exhale as you normally would. The mask is hooked up to a machine that provides oxygen and uses positive pressure to help you get rid of carbon dioxide, so your respiratory muscles don't have to work so hard to breathe. Oxygen masks are generally used when you're awake and able to assist your healthcare team in getting the mask secured properly.

Masks can be removed easily, and you retain your ability to swallow, so you don't have to worry about saliva building up or getting into your airways.

Prompt use of noninvasive ventilation has been shown to improve the outlook of COPD patients who experience respiratory failure as a result of a sudden attack. Patients who receive this treatment are less likely to die in the hospital at the time of the attack and are more likely to survive at least a year after the attack. Noninvasive ventilation also may avert the need for a breathing tube.

Invasive ventilation

Invasive ventilation is better at delivering the needed oxygen to your lungs, but it's also less comfortable and less convenient than a simple oxygen mask. A small tube called an *endotracheal tube* is placed down your throat and a hose connects it to a machine that pushes air into your lungs. This method is most often used when you're unconscious or unresponsive; it's also used in surgery.

You can't talk when you're intubated, but, if you need an endotracheal tube, you're likely to be heavily sedated anyway.

Chronic ventilation

For a small group of patients with severe COPD, there may come a time when they are no longer able to breathe without the support of mechanical ventilation. If you're in that situation, you can opt for chronic ventilation. A procedure called a *tracheotomy* creates an opening through the neck in your windpipe and a small tube that connects to a ventilator machine is inserted. This procedure usually is performed only as a last resort; according to one study, the average post-surgery life expectancy is six to seven months.

You are the final decision-maker on whether you want to receive mechanical ventilation and under what circumstances. Your doctor can help you decide when such treatment would be useful and appropriate and when you may prefer to avoid it.

Creating an Emergency Plan

Your meds can help ease the symptoms of a sudden attack, but sometimes they won't be enough, and you'll need to call your doctor or even 911 to get help. A key part of your action plan for dealing with emergencies is knowing when you can take care of your symptoms on your own and when you should seek medical help. Having a plan also can help reduce the severity and impact of sudden attacks.

You and your doctor should discuss which symptoms you should watch out for and what you can do to ease your symptoms until you can get in to see your doctor or until you receive emergency help.

Knowing your warning signs

Listening to and understanding what your body tells you is a critical component of your emergency action plan. The good news about these sudden attacks is that, even though different patients may have different warning signs, your individual warning signs likely will be the same from one attack to another and are easily recognized.

Breathlessness is the most common early warning sign, but there are others:

- ✔ Tightness in the chest
- ✔ Increased coughing
- ✔ More sputum or phlegm
- ✔ Fever

When you know the warning signs your body gives you, you can use your meds — bronchodilators and inhaled steroids — to treat your symptoms immediately. This is important because immediate self-treatment can prevent a sudden attack from getting worse, maybe even saving you a trip to the hospital.

Sudden attacks can come on at any time and in any place. Always carry your rescue inhalers with you when you leave home, and keep them in a handy place when at home.

Use *only* your rescue medications when you have an exacerbation. Your maintenance meds will not help relieve sudden, acute symptoms.

Talk with your doctor about how to use your meds in a sudden attack. If you have trouble remembering instructions, ask your doctor to write them down for you in terms you'll understand. Having an action plan in advance will help you deal more easily with a crisis when it comes.

When to call your doctor

Sometimes your bronchodilators and steroids just won't seem to do the trick. If your symptoms aren't getting any worse but aren't getting much better either, you should call your doctor within six to eight hours. Call sooner if your symptoms get worse.

If you notice a change in the amount of mucus you're coughing up, or if your mucus has a different color, is thicker than usual, or has an odor for more than a day, call your doctor. This may be a sign of a lung infection or other problem, and your doctor will need to see you to determine the right course of treatment.

You should also call your doctor within 24 hours if you have any of these symptoms:

- ✔ Swollen ankles, even after sleeping with your feet elevated
- ✔ Severe fatigue
- ✔ Waking short of breath more than once in the middle of the night

Depending on your overall health, your doctor may want you to report other symptoms as well. Ask your doctor what signs you should watch for and when he wants you to call the office.

When to call for an ambulance

Severe attacks can be life-threatening, and immediate treatment is one of the keys to survival. If you have any of the following symptoms, call 911 right away:

- ✔ **Difficulty standing, walking, or talking:** Loss of balance and difficulty walking are common symptoms of severe respiratory problems.

- ✔ **Irregular or rapid heartbeat:** Your heart may start pumping faster as it tries to deliver oxygenated blood to the rest of your body.

- ✔ **Discoloration in lips or fingernails (a gray or bluish tinge):** A bluish tinge in your lips or fingernails is a sign that oxygen levels in your blood are dangerously low.

- ✔ **Confusion, disorientation, or mental fogginess:** Slurred speech and confusion or disorientation can indicate a lack of oxygen to the brain.

- ✔ **Extreme fatigue:** Lack of adequate oxygen can make you feel extremely sleepy.

- ✔ **Difficulty breathing (and your meds don't help):** If your breathing doesn't get better with your bronchodilators and steroids, that can indicate a severe infection or other respiratory problem.

Never take extra doses of your theophylline medication when you're having a COPD crisis. High doses can make symptoms even worse and can cause other serious health problems, including irregular heartbeat and seizures.

Information you'll need

Especially in emergency situations, you probably won't see medical personnel who are familiar with your condition and history. You can help them treat you properly by preparing the information they'll need beforehand and keeping it easily accessible — in your wallet, for example, or posted on your refrigerator. Use the form on the Cheat Sheet in the front of this book to keep a current list of your medications — everything you're taking, including vitamins, nutritional supplements, over-the-counter meds, and even things like eyedrops and throat lozenges — as well as how much you take and how often you take it.

Your emergency response team also will need to know your primary doctor's name and your loved ones' contact information. If you have a healthcare proxy, advance directive, or living will, your emergency team will need to know about them as well (see "End-of-Life Planning" later in this chapter).

Keep a list of emergency contacts in your wallet and another posted on your refrigerator. This list should include not just your family members or loved ones, but also your doctor's name and phone number, the name and phone number of the hospital you usually go to, and, if applicable, a line saying you have a healthcare proxy, advance directive, or living will.

End-of-Life Planning

Understanding and treating COPD have come a long way in recent years, but it's still a progressive and eventually fatal disease. Your symptoms and overall health will get worse over time, and you may reach a point where you're unable to make healthcare decisions for yourself. As uncomfortable as it may be to think about what you want for the end of your life, talking about your options and preferences will do a lot to ease a heavy burden for you and your loved ones. You'll feel better knowing that your wishes are understood and will be carried out, and your loved ones will feel better knowing what to do when the time comes.

This isn't a one-time-only conversation. As your COPD progresses, your feelings about what treatments you want and don't want may change. It's difficult to predict what course COPD will take because there are so many other factors involved in the speed and consequences of its progression. Today's stable condition can deteriorate into a crisis tomorrow or a week from now. So it's important to start the discussion now and reopen it when you sense that circumstances may be changing.

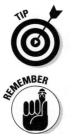

Involve your doctor in planning for your care as your COPD progresses. A good physician should be comfortable talking with you about your feelings and answering your questions.

Every patient is unique, and your doctor can only guess, based on his own experience and nationwide averages, how your COPD will progress and how long you can expect to live with the disease.

Starting the discussion

Sometimes it's easier to talk about hypothetical situations than real ones, so try thinking about what kind of treatment you would want in terms of what *may* happen:

- What if you can't breathe on your own any more?
- What if you develop pneumonia or some other serious lung infection?

- ✔ What if you have a heart attack?
- ✔ What if you have to leave your home and move to a nursing home?
- ✔ What if your chances of recovery are poor?
- ✔ What if your chances of recovery are 50-50?

Your doctor may not be able to give you a firm prognosis, but he can tell you what kinds of complications and late-stage situations are likely. This information can help you determine what you want depending on the circumstances.

Discussing whether you want life-sustaining treatments

When people have sustained sudden trauma in an accident or other incident, their treatment may include things like feeding tubes, IVs to keep them hydrated, ventilators, and other life-sustaining treatments. These treatments usually are given when the patient's condition is believed to be temporary and there is reasonable hope that she will recover.

Using these treatments in the case of chronic illnesses like late-stage cancer or COPD can be a difficult choice. On the one hand, feeding tubes, IVs, and ventilators can keep you alive and make you more comfortable. On the other, if there's little or no hope of substantial recovery, prolonging life may not be what you or your loved ones would choose.

In particular, many COPD patients fear being kept alive with mechanical ventilation. Although most patients are able to be weaned from ventilators after the cause of the crisis has been treated successfully, a few will be unable to breathe on their own again. No one can predict which patients will regain enough lung function to be taken off a ventilator and which won't. However, the more severe your COPD is and the poorer your overall health, the higher your risk of needing chronic ventilation.

You're free to choose which medical treatments you want to accept and which you want to refuse. In the absence of an advance directive or living will, emergency responders will do everything they can to keep you alive and stabilize your condition, including putting you on a ventilator.

Talk with your family about your wishes for various forms of life support. Do you want to avoid any use of mechanical ventilation? Do you want to be on a ventilator for emergencies, but have it removed if it becomes clear that you won't be able to breathe on your own again? Do you want any assistance that your medical team can give, including long-term mechanical ventilation, for as long as it takes? The decision is yours and yours alone, but your family and your doctor should know what your wishes are.

Psychologically, it's hard to decide to stop these treatments after they've begun. If you decide you want them, you may want to consider including a time limit so your doctor and your loved ones can evaluate your progress — or lack of it — and decide on next steps.

Considering resuscitation: CPR

What if you're very ill and your heart stops beating? Do you want to be resuscitated? The decision to administer CPR (short for *cardiopulmonary resuscitation*) has to be made immediately, and deciding what to do in an emergency is much easier if you've already talked about it with your family.

You need to let your doctor, home health aides, and other caregivers know what you want, too. If you're hospitalized or in a nursing home, your healthcare team can attach a Do Not Resuscitate order — commonly called a DNR — to your chart. If you're at home, your caregivers can tell emergency medical responders what your wishes are.

Putting it in writing

Different states have different rules governing *advance healthcare directives*, an umbrella term that includes living wills and healthcare proxies or surrogates. Your doctor or family lawyer should be able to tell you what the requirements are in your state; social workers and home health aides also may have this information or be able to refer you to the proper source.

Putting your wishes in writing provides some measure of assurance that your desires will be carried out if you can't make healthcare decisions for yourself. Your advance directive should include:

- A healthcare proxy or surrogate who is authorized to make healthcare decisions for you when you're unable to make them or communicate them yourself

- Instructions for your treatment in an emergency (such as a Do Not Resuscitate order)

✔ Instructions for time limits on life-sustaining treatments

✔ Instructions for evaluating the results of your treatment and determining whether you would find those results acceptable

Advance directives are most effective when they're specific. Use the what-if questions in the "Starting the discussion" section of this chapter to help you envision a variety of potential circumstances, and write down what you want in each of those situations.

Chapter 17

Helping a Loved One with COPD

*L*ike any serious chronic illness, COPD affects more than just the patient. When someone you love has COPD, you also deal with the disease physically, mentally, and emotionally. Helping out with household chores like reorganizing, housekeeping, and running errands may become more involved as the COPD progresses and your loved one needs more assistance with things like fixing meals and getting dressed. When COPD is advanced, you may even begin managing your loved one's medications and arranging visits to doctors and other services.

To do all this, you may have to rearrange your own routine and make adjustments to your own schedule. Learning about this disease can be confusing and overwhelming, especially if your loved one has other health issues that complicate his COPD.

And, emotionally, you may find yourself on an uncomfortable amusement-park ride that seems to have no end. Sadness, anger, and anxiety can raise your stress levels to alarming heights, even affecting your own physical health.

How you and your loved one approach the challenges each of you faces can set the tone for how each of you learns to live with COPD. If you're willing to help your loved one get the most out of life, and if both of you are focused on figuring out ways to manage the disease or work around it so your loved one can remain independent and active for as long as possible, you may be surprised at how well your solutions will work.

In this chapter, we give you an overview of how COPD affects your loved one and how you can help alleviate some of those effects. We also provide information on taking care of yourself; after all, you can't help your loved one if you let your own physical and mental health slip by the wayside. We talk about how you can provide practical, daily-living assistance so your loved one can preserve her independence, and we cover the things you need to know to be informed and involved in your loved one's medical care.

Brushing Up on COPD

The first thing you need to do when a loved one is diagnosed with COPD is learn as much as you can about the disease, how it's treated, and what to expect as it progresses. The more you know about it, the better prepared you are to lend as much help as possible to the COPD patient.

How COPD affects your loved one

The chapters comprising Part I of this book provide details about the causes, risk factors, and symptoms of COPD; various chapters in Part II cover tests and treatments for the disease. But, although it's important for you to have that information, equally important is understanding how your loved one's COPD is changing his life.

Part of your role in helping a loved one with COPD is understanding both the physical and emotional challenges your loved one is facing. According to an American Lung Association survey, most people with COPD say the disease puts limits on their normal level of physical activity and interferes with social activities, family activities, household chores, and sleeping. Many feel the quality of their lives is significantly diminished because of their COPD, and women are especially likely to feel this way.

All these limits, coupled with the chronic and progressive nature of COPD, can make the person with COPD feel hopeless and depressed. Feeling as though you're never going to feel better is a bleak situation to be in, and worrying about becoming a burden on a spouse or other loved ones only adds to the stress.

How your loved one's COPD affects you

Depending on your situation, you may find yourself becoming a combination of nurse, physical therapist, gofer, and counselor. If you live with your loved one, your stress levels may skyrocket as you take on all these extra roles and responsibilities. And even if you aren't dealing with it in the same home, you may find yourself overtired physically, overwhelmed mentally, and overtaxed emotionally.

Taking care of yourself

You can't take good care of anyone else if you don't take care of yourself first. Stress and lack of rest can make you more vulnerable to illness and emotional crises, which severely limits your ability to help your loved one.

Follow these tips to make your role as caregiver a little more bearable for everyone:

- **Make sure you get enough rest.** If you have trouble sleeping, consult your doctor about your options.

- **Let yourself take the easy route whenever possible.** Take advantage of technologies and tools that allow your loved one to be more independent (see Chapter 14).

- **Allow others to help you help your loved one.** You don't have to do it all the time.

- **Build some time for yourself into your schedule.** You're doing a difficult job, and you deserve regular breaks to live your own life.

- **Keep tabs on your emotional health.** If you have signs of depression, anxiety attacks, overwhelming grief, or other issues, seek help.

Because COPD is preventable in many cases, it's easy to blame the patient for the illness, especially if he is (or was) a long-term smoker. Feeling angry at your loved one for not taking better care of himself is normal, but try not to let your anger get in the way of helping your loved one manage life with COPD.

Part of taking care of yourself may involve taking a break from caregiving now and then. Explore hiring a sitter or enrolling your loved one in an adult day-care program for at least a few hours each week to give yourself some time off.

Coping with your grief

When a loved one is chronically ill, it's not uncommon for the grieving process to start immediately and last throughout the remainder of your loved one's life and, of course, her death and the aftermath. Ignoring these feelings can add to your stress level, which can affect your physical health. Remember that you and your loved one are both grieving the loss of your lives before COPD, even as you try to cope with life with COPD.

Very likely, your grief will be unpredictable. You'll have good days and bad, just as your loved one will. The trick is enjoying the times when grief fades into the background and dealing with the times when grief sneaks up on you.

Here are some tips that have worked for others in similar situations:

- ✔ **Take time to be by yourself.** Being alone gives you time to think about and process your feelings in the way that works for you. Some people need to release their emotions through a good cry; others need to pray; still others find that going for a walk or taking a nap helps.

- ✔ **Get help from others.** Whether by giving you a break from your caregiving responsibilities or just by joining you for coffee or a visit, letting other people into your life can make you feel better.

- ✔ **Stick to a routine.** Routines help you ensure that you get enough rest and exercise and that you eat as healthfully as you can. They also provide a measure of comfort; when some areas of your life are in a period of upheaval, the elements of your routine can act as small islands of normalcy.

Finding support

Caring for a chronically ill loved one can make you feel isolated. The care itself takes so much time that, often, you feel you can't spare even an hour to get out in the world and find out what's going on, and you may feel envious of people who don't have similar demands to cope with.

Fortunately, there are lots of places to turn for help, information, and moral support from people who have been in your shoes and people who are there now. Just knowing you're not alone can be a tremendous boost to your spirits. Often these groups have information and tips to make your life — and your loved one's life — a little easier.

Start by ordering Beth Israel Medical Center's *Caregiver Resource Directory,* which includes advice for caring for a loved one and for yourself. Order online at www.netofcare.org/crd/resource_form.asp. Best of all, it's free of charge.

Here are some useful Web sites to get you started:

- ✔ **AARP (www.aarp.org/families):** In the "Family, Home, and Legal" section of the AARP Web site, you can find message boards where you can communicate with other people going through the same kinds of struggles you are — they may or may not have loved ones with COPD, but the issues and feelings they're coping with may be very similar to your own. The site also has information about a variety of topics, including home care and financing for long-term care.

- ✔ **Caregiver.com (www.caregiver.com):** This Web site has a discussion forum, back issues of *Today's Caregiver* magazine, and information on conferences you can attend to learn more. A one-year subscription to

Today's Caregiver costs $18 for U.S. addresses ($26 for Canadian addresses); a two-year subscription costs $32 U.S. ($50 Canada). You can subscribe through the Web site or by calling 800-829-2734.

✔ **COPD-Support, Inc. (www.copd-support.com):** This is a support, education, and information site for people with COPD and their caregivers.

✔ **Emphysema Foundation for Our Right to Survive (www.emphysema. net):** This is an organization of patients and family caregivers providing information and resources.

✔ **Family Caregiver Alliance (www.caregiver.org):** This site offers online support for family caregivers. *Note:* It also is available in Spanish.

✔ **National Family Caregivers Association (www.nfcacares.org):** This organization provides education and support for people who care for chronically ill loved ones. Topics include improving communication with doctors, self-advocacy for caregivers, and tips for family caregivers.

✔ **Well Spouse Association (www.wellspouse.org):** This site lists regional activities and publications for spouse caregivers, as well as local groups and e-mail networks.

If you don't have Internet access, check with your local library. Many of even the smallest libraries have computers for the public to use. Your librarian also can help you find other resources.

Your loved one's doctor, counselor, or social worker may be able to provide helpful tips on making your role easier. He also may be able to refer you to local support groups for caregivers.

Understanding the Treatment

Proper use of COPD medications is critical to managing the disease well, but patients can find the instructions confusing. One of the ways you can provide practical assistance for your loved one is by understanding her treatment plan.

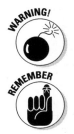

Federal law restricts sharing healthcare information without the express consent of the patient. Your loved one may have to sign an authorization form before her doctor or other healthcare providers will talk with you about her condition or treatment.

Because there is no cure for COPD, treatment focuses on managing symptoms and slowing down the progression of the disease.

Commonly prescribed drugs

COPD treatment plans depend on a number of variables: the severity of the COPD, other health issues that may complicate treatment, the patient's reaction to typical COPD meds, and so on. Treatment plans also change as the disease progresses and when the patient experiences suddenly worsening symptoms (called *acute exacerbations*) or an infection. Chapter 8 has detailed information about drug treatments for COPD.

Bronchodilators

Bronchodilators help relax and widen the airways so getting air in and out is easier. Some are effective within minutes and last for a few hours; others take longer to start working but last longer and only have to be taken once or twice a day. Many COPD patients use a combination of short- and long-acting bronchodilators.

Steroids

Certain kinds of steroids (not the kind that have caused scandals in professional and Olympic sports) are generally prescribed to help a COPD patient get over an acute exacerbation or infection. Long-term steroid treatment is uncommon in patients with mild or moderate COPD, but steroids are sometimes prescribed for patients with severe or late-stage COPD. Steroids help reduce swelling and mucus production., which is why they're often used to treat sudden attacks. There also is evidence that these kinds of steroids can help other medications work better.

Antibiotics, flu shots, and vaccines

Antibiotics are prescribed when a COPD patient has a bacterial infection — not a viral infection, because antibiotics are ineffective against viruses. People with COPD are more likely to succumb to colds and the flu, so most doctors recommend an annual flu shot for their COPD patients. A pneumonia vaccination is recommended every five years.

Oxygen therapy

Home oxygen therapy can improve quality of life for many people with severe COPD; often, it allows such patients to be more active and independent. It also can be beneficial for people with less severe COPD during certain activities like exercise or sleep.

Recommended lifestyle changes

Medications can only help manage COPD symptoms; they can't reverse the damage that's been done to the lungs or slow down the progression of the disease. So your loved one's COPD treatment plan includes specific lifestyle recommendations: Quit smoking, eat better, and exercise.

Quitting smoking

Some patients figure, when they've been diagnosed with COPD, there's no reason to quit smoking. But continuing to smoke just does more damage to the lungs, which speeds up the progression of COPD and makes it much more difficult to manage.

If your loved one has decided to quit smoking, you can help by offering both moral and practical support. Provide encouragement when needed, but don't nag; instead, express sympathy over withdrawal symptoms, confidence in your loved one's ability to overcome the addiction, and praise for the progress made so far.

Make sure there are plenty of healthy, easy-to-reach, and already-prepared snacks in the house. Make the house a smoke-free zone (you should do this anyway because secondhand smoke can harm you and your loved one) and tell smokers they must go outside to light up. And encourage your loved one to move around; taking a walk together is an easy way for both of you to get some fresh air and exercise.

Eating properly

COPD patients often need to change their diets to get enough energy without jeopardizing their overall health. You can help by learning about your loved one's nutritional requirements (see Chapter 11 for information on nutrition and weight management), making out grocery lists, and even preparing meals.

Many people with COPD find preparing meals exhausting, so they tend to rely on prepackaged foods, which may not be good for their general health or for their lung function. You can make your own prepackaged, healthy meals that can be refrigerated or frozen in single-serve containers, so all your loved one has to do is heat them up.

Drinking plenty of fluids, especially water, helps keep mucus thin, so it's easier to cough up. Check with your loved one's doctor to make sure there aren't any restrictions on fluid intake, and, if there aren't, make sure your loved gets lots of fluids every day.

Lots of variables may affect your loved one's ideal fluid intake, so ask your loved one's doctor for recommendations. Remember, too, that, although water is great, not all fluid *must* be straight water; tea, juice, coffee, and soda may be appropriate alternatives.

People with COPD often have poor appetites because digestion takes so much energy. Eating smaller meals more often can help your loved one get the calories and nutrients he needs without leading to feelings of exhaustion.

Although fruits and vegetables are good sources of nutrients, they can cause gas or bloating, which can make breathing more difficult. Don't urge your loved one to eat foods that may cause these symptoms, even if the foods are generally healthy.

Exercising

Physical activity is critical to making the most of the lung function your loved one has and to help ease symptoms of breathlessness and fatigue. Exercise also is a proven mood brightener, so it can help your loved one physically and emotionally.

Nearly everyone finds it easier to stick with an exercise regimen if there's someone else to do it with. You can help your loved one get the exercise she needs by taking walks or water aerobics classes together, or even just by standing by while she does a few minutes on a treadmill or stationary bike.

Looking At Other Ways You Can Help

You can do a surprising number of things to help your loved one feel more comfortable, both physically and emotionally. Make the time to talk about your loved one's goals and challenges, and ask what he thinks would help. Your loved one may have suggestions that you (and we) may never think of.

That said, there are common areas where you can help your loved one preserve a sense of independence and interest in life, and we cover them in this section.

Arranging outings

Cabin fever affects even healthy people who can't get outside because of the weather or other factors. Your loved one may experience severe bouts of cabin fever if COPD limits his ability to get out of the house. If you can make arrangements for your loved one to go out occasionally, chances are, both of you will feel better.

Going out takes a lot of energy when you have COPD. Any outing — lunch, for instance, or going to a movie or concert — may require your planning and assistance. Just going to the grocery store can be an exhausting chore. You can help by making a shopping list in advance and going with your loved one to the store. Choose times when the store is apt to be less crowded, and, if your loved one has trouble walking, get a motorized cart for her to use.

People with COPD often move more slowly than the rest of us, so include extra time when you're planning an outing. If time is tight, it may be less stressful for both of you if you do an errand yourself or if you postpone the activity to a day when you aren't so rushed.

Helping with household chores

Having a clean house is not just a morale booster; it's better for your loved one's health. Dust, mildew, and other airborne irritants can make breathing more difficult. They even can prompt sudden attacks that are always scary and sometimes life-threatening.

But keeping up with the housework can be beyond the energy limits of people with COPD. Dusting, vacuuming, cleaning the bathroom and kitchen, and even doing laundry can be daunting when you can't breathe properly. If you don't have time to do these kinds of chores yourself, perhaps you can pay for a cleaning person to come in every week or two to do the cleaning for your loved one. If that isn't feasible, see if other family members can help with these chores.

Adapting the COPD home

Lifting, bending, and walking all become more difficult for your loved one as COPD gets worse. Reorganizing the kitchen, bathroom, bedroom, and even living room can help your loved one get around more easily and do more on his own. (Chapter 14 has tips for making changes around the home to accommodate the physical limitations that COPD imposes.)

Helping find new interests

COPD may limit your loved one's ability to do things she used to enjoy, and that loss easily can lead to depression and a lack of interest in life. You may be able to ease these effects by helping your loved one discover new interests that aren't so physically taxing.

It may take some creativity to find activities your loved one can do. The easiest first step is to think in terms of scale. If keeping up an outdoor garden is too strenuous, for instance, you could help your loved one set up a small indoor garden that doesn't require as much maintenance or labor.

A computer with Internet access can be a great boon to people whose mobility is limited. Your loved one can use it to keep up with current events, research interests, play games, and even make new friends in online communities.

Keeping your loved one comfortable

There are various techniques you can use to alleviate the physical discomfort of COPD. Simple things like making sure your loved one has a comfortable place to sit are important to overall quality of life and sense of well-being.

You also can ask to be trained in techniques like chest or back tapping to help relieve congestion and other symptoms. Talk to your loved one's doctor, home health aide, or physical therapist about which techniques to use and how to do them.

Paying attention to emotional health

One of your roles as caregiver is to keep tabs on your loved one's emotional health. It's normal for your loved one to feel sad or down in the dumps occasionally. You want to watch for sustained periods of listlessness, sadness, or lack of interest. These can be signs of depression, which can be treated. Encourage your loved one to talk about how he feels. If you have concerns about your loved one's emotional health, talk to his doctor.

Getting Involved in Medical Care

Even if your loved one's COPD is in the mild or moderate stage, you should make an effort to meet your loved one's healthcare team so you can better help implement the treatment plan and know what to expect as the disease progresses. As COPD gets worse, you'll likely play an ever-growing role in helping your loved one manage symptoms, make lifestyle changes, and deal with crises. The earlier you get involved, the more comfortable you'll feel as your caregiving role expands.

Talking with the medical team

The doctors and other healthcare professionals who treat your loved one can also give you valuable guidance on how to help. In the beginning, you'll want to know what your loved one needs and how you can help make sure she gets what she needs. As the disease progresses, the healthcare team can help you keep things in perspective by letting you know how your loved one's condition has changed and what it will mean for both of you, as well as what to expect from this point on.

If your loved one has a social worker or case manager, that person can help you figure out rules for Medicare and Medicaid. He also can provide information about services and facilities, like adult day-care centers, that may be appropriate for your situation.

Getting a prognosis

Whenever someone gets a diagnosis of a serious illness, the first question that comes to mind is, "How long will I (or he or she) live?" There's nothing wrong with asking that question, but be prepared for your doctor to say the equivalent of, "I don't know." COPD is a difficult disease to predict. Some people remain stable for very long periods before they experience a real decline in health status or even episodes where their symptoms are suddenly worse. Others may show signs of the disease's progression much more quickly.

There is a tendency, also, to consider a prognosis firm once it is given. But, especially in COPD, there are so many other factors that can influence your loved one's overall health that the prognosis can easily change over time.

The "How long?" conversation is one you should revisit periodically with the doctor, especially if you have questions about your loved one's treatment, if your loved one has other health issues that can affect his COPD or quality of life, and when your loved one's condition changes.

Understanding what changes mean

When your loved one's condition or treatment plan changes, it's a good time to talk to the doctor about what you can expect now. This helps you keep changes in perspective and protect yourself — and your loved one — from having unrealistic or unreasonable expectations.

Here are some questions you may want to ask:

- ✔ Does this change in condition or treatment change the patient's prognosis?
- ✔ Are there other changes or complications we should expect?
- ✔ What can we do to avoid or minimize complications?
- ✔ What is the best we can hope for now?
- ✔ What is the worst-case scenario?
- ✔ What usually happens with COPD patients in similar conditions?

Your loved one's primary doctor may not know the answers to these questions; much depends on how much experience he's had with following COPD patients through to death. If the primary doctor can't answer these questions, you may want to ask them of the pulmonologist, who should have more experience in the myriad ways COPD can affect individuals.

Understanding the instructions

COPD medications are key to managing symptoms and maintaining physical function for a better quality of life. But many COPD patients find the instructions for taking their meds bewildering. You can help make sure your loved one is taking medications properly by making sure you understand all the instructions and how to use devices like inhalers and nebulizers. (Chapter 8 has information and illustrations on taking medications properly.)

Research has shown that instructions on prescriptions are easily misunderstood and that skipping doses or taking medications improperly can be deadly. If you don't understand how your loved one is supposed to take medications, ask the doctor, nurse, or pharmacist for clearer instructions. Don't give up until you're sure you know what your loved one is supposed to do.

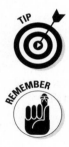

If you don't live with your loved one, you can help make sure she's taking medications properly by calling every day and asking which meds she's taken and when. Make a chart with the name, dosage, and frequency (once a day, morning and evening, and so on) or the time it should be taken and check off each med that has been taken.

Inhalers are medicines, too, and they have to be used correctly to give the best results. Include inhaled medicines on your chart and make sure your loved one knows how to use inhalers properly.

Providing transportation

One of your most common duties as a caregiver, even when COPD is in its less severe stages, probably will be providing transportation to and from doctor's appointments. It won't always be convenient, but it is important that your loved one see the doctor regularly, even if there has been no change in his symptoms or overall health. Besides, if you're giving your loved one a ride to the doctor's office, you have another opportunity to talk to the doctor about your questions and concerns.

Coping with Crises

Sudden worsening of symptoms and panic attacks that result in shortness of breath can be frightening both for the person experiencing them and for you to watch. Having an emergency action plan in place can help you stay calm when a crisis does arise, and if you're calm, your loved one is more likely to calm down more quickly.

Chapter 16 discusses creating a plan for dealing with emergencies and knowing when to put your plan into action. It's important that both you and your loved one know when you should call the doctor and when you should dial 911.

Your loved one's doctor probably has prescribed "stand-by" medications for dealing with sudden onset of severe symptoms. Make sure you always have these meds on hand and know how to use them appropriately.

Whom to call

Keep the following information next to the phone, or someplace where it's handy and won't get lost:

- ✔ Primary doctor's name
- ✔ Primary doctor's office number
- ✔ Primary doctor's answering service or pager number
- ✔ Alternate doctor's name — this may be a partner in the primary doctor's office or your loved one's pulmonologist or other healthcare provider
- ✔ Alternate doctor's office number
- ✔ Alternate doctor's answering service or pager number

You also should know which hospital your loved one should go to, and you should have phone numbers for the ambulance service and emergency rooms posted near the phone or in some other convenient spot.

When to call

Not all symptoms warrant a call for an ambulance, or even to the doctor's office. Mild attacks can usually be treated at home with the meds your loved one already has. Using these meds immediately sometimes can clear up symptoms altogether; even in more severe attacks, immediate treatment with your loved one's regular meds can keep a sudden attack from getting worse.

If symptoms don't get better within a few hours, though, you probably should call the doctor. She may recommend different medications or dosages and may want to see your loved one to test for infection.

Call the doctor if your loved one has:

- A harder time breathing during normal activities
- Wheezing or increased wheezing during normal activities
- An increase in mucus production
- A change in mucus, such as an odor or change in color
- Chest pain with coughing
- Swelling in the extremities, particularly the ankles and feet
- Severe fatigue

Call for an ambulance if your loved one has:

- Difficulty standing or walking
- Slurred speech or difficulty talking
- Gray or blue tinge in the lips or fingernails
- Difficulty breathing (and meds aren't helping)
- Trouble concentrating or symptoms of disorientation or confusion

Keep paper and pens by the phone so you can write down instructions you get from the doctor's office or ambulance dispatcher. If you don't understand the instructions, ask questions until you do.

What medical personnel need to know

When you call the doctor or the ambulance, they'll need to know what symptoms are causing your concern, how long it's been since the symptoms appeared, what medications your loved one is taking, and when the meds were last taken. Being prepared with this information can help you stay calm and follow the instructions you're given to care for your loved one until you can get to the doctor's office or until emergency personnel arrive.

Make a copy of the medication form on the Cheat Sheet in the front of this book (or just tear it out of the book), and keep it next to the phone or on the refrigerator at your loved one's home. Your calls to the doctor's office and emergency services will be much less stressful if you have a medication list all ready to refer to.

If you have any questions about when it's appropriate to call the doctor or an ambulance, ask your loved one's doctor for guidance. Make a list of symptoms to watch for and keep it with the medications and emergency contact list so you have all the information you need in one place.

Part V
The Part of Tens

The 5th Wave   By Rich Tennant

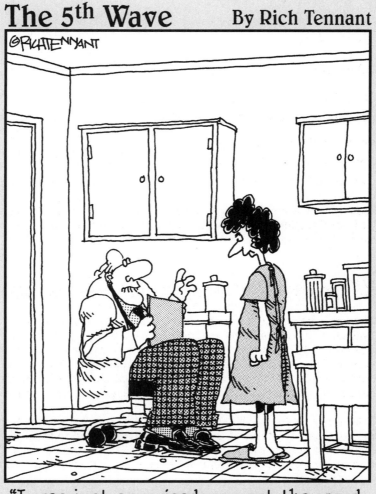

"I was just surprised you put the word
'marriage' next to the question asking
if you suffered from a chronic condition."

In this part . . .

COPD can be overwhelming because it affects so many areas of your life. Our Part of Tens is devoted to simple ways to deal with the disease on a daily basis.

Here you find ten things to avoid so your COPD symptoms don't get worse, ten myths about COPD, ten strategies for coping with COPD in both the short and long term, and ten health factors you should keep an eye on when you have COPD.

Chapter 18

Ten Things to Avoid if You Have COPD

In This Chapter

▶ Identifying triggers that can make your symptoms worse

▶ Understanding why these things can be harmful

▶ Finding tricks to deal with the triggers you can't avoid

*W*hen you have COPD, you have to be especially vigilant in monitoring your health, and this means monitoring your surroundings as well. Conditions that are nothing more than minor irritants to healthy people can cause you serious problems. In this chapter, we present ten common triggers that can make your COPD symptoms worse and explain why you should do your best to avoid them.

Of course, you can't always get away from things that may trigger an acute attack or just generally make you feel crummy. So we also provide some tips for minimizing the impact of these things if you just can't avoid them altogether.

Smoke

When it comes to COPD, smoke is public enemy number one. Smoke from cigarettes, pipes, wood stoves, or campfires can make it harder for you to breathe. Prolonged exposure can cause permanent damage to your lungs, heart, and other organs, too.

If you smoke, of course, the first step you need to take is to quit. (Chapter 10 covers smoking, what it does to you, and how to quit.) Quitting now is the best way to slow the progression of your COPD; your immune system will be better able to fight off infection, your heart will work better, and you'll preserve whatever lung function you have left.

Staying away from secondhand smoke is important, too, because it's just as harmful to your lungs as smoking yourself. Ask friends and family members who smoke to refrain from lighting up around you. Make your home a smoke-free zone and insist that smokers go outside when they want a cigarette. Don't allow smoking in your car, either; the confined space, even with a window cracked, exposes you to a great deal of secondhand smoke.

Smoke from wood stoves and campfires can cause problems for you, especially if it drifts directly toward you. If you have COPD, avoid using wood stoves as a heating source, because fine particles in the air can irritate your lungs. If you can't avoid using or being near a wood stove, try positioning a fan to direct airflow from the stove away from you. Use dry, seasoned wood or pellets to minimize creation of smoke.

Position yourself upwind of campfires, and keep a handkerchief or bandana handy to cover your nose and mouth if the wind shifts unexpectedly.

Fumes

All kinds of fumes can irritate your airways and lead to severe shortness of breath and other symptoms. Paint and paint thinner, weedkillers and insecticides, gasoline, even household cleaning products, air fresheners, perfume, and cooking odors can cause problems for you.

Here are some steps you can take to minimize your exposure to some fumes:

- Make sure painting or bug spraying in your house is done when you're away.

- When you return home after painting or spraying has been done, open the windows and turn on fans to get the air moving and cleared of fumes.

- Ask friends or family members to apply weedkillers and insecticides for you, and stay indoors with the windows closed if you're home when they do it.

- Buy paints, insecticides, weedkillers, and even household chemicals in small quantities. These products can give off fumes even when they're being stored. If you have to store paints and so on, put them in the garage or an outdoor shed to keep the fumes from accumulating in your home.

- Ask friends or relatives to fill your car with gas for you. If you have to do it yourself, start the pump and then get back in the car with the windows up to minimize your exposure to gasoline fumes.

Sliding into and out of a car can cause static electricity, which can trigger a fire when you touch the gas nozzle. So after you get out of the car, and before you touch the gas nozzle again, touch something metal — your car door, for example — to discharge that static electricity.

✔ Look for unscented cleaning products, including dish soap, laundry detergent, and dryer sheets. If you're very sensitive to perfumes, buy unscented bath soaps and shampoos, too.

✔ Avoid scented air fresheners. Instead, look for unscented varieties of sprays and candles.

✔ Use the exhaust fans in your kitchen and bathroom to help remove odors from cooking and cleaning.

✔ Keep a window near the stove cracked, even in cold weather, to help ventilate the kitchen while you're cooking.

High Pollution Areas

Crowded thoroughfares and traffic jams are horrible places for COPD sufferers. Even for healthy people, the air in these areas can be next to unbreathable. Exhaust and smog can cause acute irritation and inflammation of your airways.

What if you live in a city, where it's nearly impossible to avoid car exhaust and smog? Take precautions when you go out. If you're not comfortable wearing a dust mask, try wearing a light scarf; you can pull it up to cover your nose and mouth when the pollution starts to make breathing difficult for you.

Watch the weather forecast, too. When the pollution index is particularly bad, or when high ozone warnings are issued, your best bet is to stay home in an air-conditioned room.

You tend to breathe in through your mouth when you exercise, because you need to draw in more air when you're exerting yourself. Avoid exercising outdoors when pollution is bad or ozone warnings are in effect; breathing through your mouth means you'll inhale more of these irritants.

Windy, Dusty Days

Just like pollution, wind and dust can make it hard for you to catch your breath. If you don't have to go out on days like this, stay home. You may want to keep your windows closed and the air conditioner on, too, because wind can easily kick dust, pollen, and other irritants into your home.

If you can't avoid going outdoors when it's windy and dusty, wear a dust mask or scarf so you can keep dust from getting into your lungs.

Very Cold Air

Extremely cold air causes your airways to tighten up, which makes it harder to expel air. Eventually, the air trapped in your lungs can make you feel like you can't get enough air *in*. When you have COPD, this tightening just worsens the symptoms you already have, making you feel even more short of breath. For some people, the air doesn't even have to be extremely cold to cause breathing difficulties.

If cold air bothers you and you can't stay indoors all the time, here are some options for you:

- ✔ **Breathe through your nose.** This warms and moisturizes the air, making it more comfortable to inhale.

- ✔ **Wear a cold-air mask when you go outside.** Cold-air masks are available at most drugstores in colder climates. You also can find them online at sites like www.icanbreathe.com.

- ✔ **Wear a face mask or scarf that covers your nose and mouth.** This helps warm and moisturize the air before you inhale.

High Humidity

Humidity is one of those tricky factors when you have COPD. Super-dry air can make breathing difficult — but so can super-moist air. Generally, humidity of around 40 percent is comfortable for most COPD patients.

In the summer months, though, depending on where you live, humidity levels can reach 70 percent, 80 percent, even 90 percent or higher. Combine high humidity with high temperatures, and trying to breathe can feel like trying to suck ice cream through a swizzle stick.

When heat and humidity bother you, air conditioning is your best friend. Air conditioning cools the air by removing some moisture from it, bringing humidity down to a comfortable level. If you don't have air conditioning, use a fan to keep the air circulating, and avoid exerting yourself as much as possible.

As your COPD progresses, fans may give you a psychological as well as a physical benefit: They can make you feel like you're getting more air flow, which can help you relax and perhaps prevent panic breathing.

Heavy Meals

The more you eat, the bigger your stomach gets, which can make you feel like you don't have room to expand your lungs. Bulky foods that cause gas — like fried, spicy foods or certain fruits and vegetables — can increase your discomfort.

Digestion takes a great deal of energy, and the more there is to digest, the more energy it takes. Smaller meals are less tiring to eat and digest than large meals. Resting before and after eating can make meals less wearing, too. But don't lie down after eating; your full stomach can put pressure on your chest cavity so you feel like it's harder to breathe.

The process of digesting carbohydrates creates more carbon dioxide in your body, so you may feel more short of breath than usual. Staying away from breads and pasta can make breathing easier during and after meals.

Keep portions small and try to eat foods that don't fill you up too much. Eat slowly: Take small bites, put your utensils down between bites, and chew each bite thoroughly to avoid possible choking.

Don't drink liquids right before or during a meal. Liquids, especially carbonated drinks like soda, fill you up and can cause gas. Save your beverage for after your meal.

High Sodium Content

Salt makes your body retain water, which can make you feel bloated and uncomfortable. Water retention also can make your heart work harder because it increases blood pressure, and that extra heart work can make you feel even more short of breath.

To keep your salt and sodium consumption under control, follow these tips:

✔ Don't add salt to foods while cooking.

✔ Try to use salt-free seasonings in your recipes.

✔ When eating, always taste foods before adding salt. If necessary, remove the salt shaker from the table.

✔ When choosing prepared foods, look for ones with 300 milligrams of sodium or less per serving.

Sick People

When you have COPD, you're more susceptible to colds, flu, pneumonia, and other infections, because your immune system isn't as robust. This means you need to take extra care in avoiding situations where you may pick up a bug. Friends and family should keep their distance when they have colds, sore throats, or other signs of illness. Children, in particular, often pass along respiratory infections.

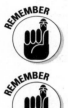

Your best defense, especially during cold and flu season, is to wash your hands frequently. Germs lurk virtually everywhere and are easily transferred from your hands to your eyes, nose, and mouth. Washing your hands often can kill a huge majority of these germs and protect you from catching whatever's going around.

Make sure you get your annual flu shot and a pneumonia vaccine every five years.

Overexertion

Too much activity, even if it's pleasant activity, can make you tired and short of breath. It also makes your heart work harder and can affect your appetite — a critical consideration when you have COPD, because you need to eat to keep your energy levels up.

Don't be afraid to do activities you enjoy, but do be smart about taking part in those activities. Learn what your limitations are and respect them. Take frequent rest breaks so you don't overtire yourself, and resist the urge to push yourself beyond reasonable limits. If others push you to do more than you should, stand up for yourself — after all, you know better than anyone else what you can and cannot do.

Chapter 19

Ten Myths about COPD

Ten years ago, maybe even five years ago, most people had never heard of COPD. It was considered a smoker's disease (when it was considered at all), so those who had it often received little sympathy or empathy for their disease or its debilitating effects. This isn't entirely fair to smokers who develop COPD, because, until relatively recently, smoking was both socially acceptable and prominently promoted.

When COPD is caused by smoking, it *is* a preventable disease. But not all the blame for COPD can be laid at tobacco's door, and, even for COPD patients who smoke or used to smoke, the disease warrants a great deal more understanding than it gets. In this chapter, we take on ten of the most common misconceptions about COPD and tell you the truth about this disease.

COPD Is a Rare Condition

Twelve million Americans are currently diagnosed with COPD, and another 12 million are believed to have COPD but haven't been properly diagnosed. According to the National Heart, Lung, and Blood Institute (part of the National Institutes of Health), someone dies from COPD in the United States every four minutes — that's 120,000 deaths a year, making COPD the fourth leading cause of death in the United States.

Although COPD currently ranks behind heart disease, cancer, and stroke as a leading cause of death for Americans, it is the only one in the top four with numbers that are rising. As COPD becomes better understood and better diagnosed, disabilities and deaths attributed to it will continue to increase.

COPD Is a Man's Disease

At one time, conventional wisdom asserted that COPD strikes white men in their 60s who smoke or used to smoke. Today, women are more likely than men to be diagnosed with COPD, and they're more likely to begin suffering the effects of the disease in their 50s or earlier. Part of the reason for this is that, while the number of male smokers has declined over the past several years, the number of female smokers has increased. Plus, nonsmoking women are more likely than nonsmoking men to develop COPD.

Women also suffer more severe forms of COPD than men do, for reasons that aren't yet fully understood. Women who have COPD also are more likely than male COPD patients to suffer from depression, to need continual oxygen therapy earlier than men, and to describe their quality of life as "poor." And more women than men die from COPD each year.

COPD also may be underdiagnosed in black men and women.

Only Smokers Get COPD

In nearly nine out of ten COPD cases, current or former smoking is, indeed, the culprit. Smoking absolutely increases your risk of developing COPD. But at least one of every ten COPD patients has never smoked. These people may have been exposed to secondhand smoke or other harmful fumes, either at home or on the job, or they may have a rare genetic disorder that almost inevitably leads to emphysema and COPD. HIV also can cause emphysema in nonsmokers.

And while smoking is the number-one risk for COPD, not all smokers will become COPD patients. In fact, only about 20 percent of current or former smokers will eventually develop this disease, and this group typically has a significant smoking history. We don't yet know why COPD strikes such a small fraction of smokers, but researchers suspect some genetic factor may be in play.

Quitting Smoking Can Cure COPD

Nothing can cure COPD. But because smoking is so harmful to your body in general and to your lungs in particular, kicking the habit is the first thing you should do and one of the best things you can do to slow the progression of COPD. Every time you inhale cigarette smoke, you also inhale toxic fumes that can be absorbed into your bloodstream and tiny particles that sink to the bottom of your lungs and form tar. This just adds to the damage your lungs already have and eventually will make your COPD symptoms worse and harder to treat.

We're not saying it's easy to quit smoking; we know better. You have to overcome not only the physical addiction to nicotine but the psychological addiction to the act of smoking itself. It requires determination, commitment, and perseverance to quit. Perseverance is especially important: By some estimates, the average smoker makes seven serious attempts at quitting before finally becoming tobacco-free. (See Chapter 10 for detailed information on why smoking is so addictive and for ways to kick the habit. Also check out *Quitting Smoking For Dummies,* by David Brizer, MD [Wiley].)

Tossing the cigarettes won't cure your COPD, but it will decrease the rate of damage to your lungs and make it easier to manage the disease.

When You Have COPD, There's No Reason to Quit Smoking

Some people believe, mistakenly, that if they've been diagnosed with COPD, they may as well keep on smoking. After all, they reason, the damage is done, I'm doomed to a shortened life anyway, so why should I give up one of the things I enjoy?

The fact is that quitting smoking plays a huge role in slowing down the progression of COPD. True, quitting won't undo the damage that has already been done, but every puff of cigarette smoke just adds to the damage your lungs have suffered. People with COPD who continue to smoke often never get to feel better; their life expectancy is significantly shorter, and their quality of life gets progressively worse at a much faster rate than it does for COPD patients who do quit smoking.

Your doctor has lots of new options to help you quit smoking. But, as always, you have to *want* to quit; without that desire, any smoking cessation method you try is bound to fail.

Children Get COPD

COPD develops over the course of many years, the product of risky behaviors like smoking; environmental exposures at home, at work, or out in the neighborhood; and, sometimes, genetic disposition. Children do not get COPD, although children who have asthma or numerous lung infections may be at greater risk of developing the disease as adults. Children who are exposed to secondhand smoke, and young asthmatics who smoke themselves, increase their risks of developing many lung diseases, including COPD, later in life.

COPD Is Only a Problem When Symptoms Are Severe

Severe COPD symptoms can be life-threatening, but that doesn't mean that COPD's less serious symptoms have no impact.

COPD interferes with overall quality of life by making you feel too tired, too short of breath, or too weak to do the things you'd like to do. For many people with COPD, the onset of the disease is so subtle that the signs are mistaken for other things — normal aging, gaining weight, being out of shape. The inability to breathe well leads you to take the elevator instead of attempting the stairs. It makes you beg off when friends or family members want you to go out with them. It prompts you to bring in just two bags of groceries at a time instead of four, or to get someone else to do it for you.

Over time, you find your activity level sharply reduced, and you may not even know why. *Remember:* Half of adults who are believed to have COPD have not been diagnosed. Without treatment, you're bound to feel worse, and the worse you feel, the more your quality of life suffers.

COPD Can't Be Treated

COPD is incurable, but that's not the same thing as untreatable. Medications can help open your airways and make breathing easier for you; oxygen therapy can counter feelings of being short of breath, weak, or lightheaded. An appropriate exercise program and a diet that makes sense for you and your overall health can help you feel better and give you energy to do at least some of the things you want to do.

A diagnosis of COPD doesn't mean you have to sit in your easy chair and wait to die. By working with your healthcare team — your primary doctor, your pulmonologist, your dietitian, your rehabilitation staff, and your counselor — you can learn how to live with your disease and still get as much out of life as possible.

When You Go on Oxygen, You Have to Be on It Forever

Oxygen therapy has proven to be highly beneficial to some COPD patients, and it's the only treatment known to prolong survival, but strong negative associations with oxygen treatment persist. Some people believe that oxygen therapy is a last-ditch effort to prolong a patient's life; others believe that people on oxygen therapy are confined to their homes, unable to travel or even go to the grocery store.

Sometimes, COPD patients are able to discontinue their oxygen therapy after other treatments have taken effect. This weaning from oxygen takes time, and it isn't appropriate for every patient. Much depends on all the other factors that play a role in your therapy and prognosis.

But the mere use of oxygen therapy does not need to trap you in your home. Several options for portable oxygen therapy exist, so you can take a stroll, go to a concert, and do errands as much as you want. With advance planning, you can even travel while on oxygen therapy.

People with COPD Can't Live Normal Lives

Because COPD affects so many aspects of your life, it's easy to feel overwhelmed. But lots of people with COPD are able to enjoy many of their favorite activities. You have to take care of yourself by exercising and eating properly, following your medication schedule, and, probably, making some adjustments in your daily routine to take advantage of your high-energy times and conserve your energy when you don't have much of it.

This is why setting treatment goals with your healthcare team is so important. You decide what's important to you — if you want to be able to continue gardening, for example, or to go out to eat with friends once a week — and you and your healthcare team figure out the best way to help you achieve your goals. With the proper care and attitude, you can continue to live a "normal" life long after your doctor utters the term *COPD*.

Chapter 20

Ten Strategies for Coping with COPD

Medications can do a lot to help you breathe easier and feel better when you have COPD, but there's a lot more you can do to help yourself. Here are our top ten strategies for managing your COPD and getting the most out of life.

See Your Doctor Regularly

Don't ditch your doctor's appointment just because you happen to be feeling okay. Keeping an eye on your lung function is important, so see your physician at least twice a year. Look at it this way: If you're feeling better, don't you want to be able to brag to your doctor about it? (It'll make your doctor feel good, too.)

At every doctor's visit, go over your medications, including over-the-counter drugs and any vitamins or nutritional or herbal supplements you're taking. If you experience any side effects, mention them to your doctor. He may be able to adjust your dosage or try a different medication to minimize unpleasant side effects.

Also talk to your doctor about getting a pneumonia vaccination and a yearly flu shot. When you have COPD, you're more susceptible to respiratory infections and complications, so doing what you can to protect yourself is important.

Set Goals for Your Daily Activity Level

COPD can put severe limits on what you're able to do every day, and those limitations can make you feel discouraged or depressed. When you set goals for what you'd like to do, you give yourself a better sense of control, which helps fight those get-me-down feelings.

Here are some things to consider in setting your goals:

✔ **Be realistic.** COPD is an exhausting disease, and you may not have the energy to do what you used to do in a typical day. Choose the activities that are most important to you, and focus on accomplishing them. A reasonable daily goal is getting out of the house for a stroll, for instance — not spending the day hiking in the mountains.

✔ **Break big jobs into smaller pieces.** If one of your goals is to get your closet organized, make today's goal organizing your shoes or skirts. Tomorrow you can concentrate on organizing your slacks, and the top shelf can be your project for the day after.

✔ **Keep your long-term goals in mind.** If you want to be able to exercise for 20 minutes a day eventually, set smaller daily exercise goals that will move you toward your larger goal. Maybe you've been exercising 5 minutes a day for a while; today, your goal can be to exercise for 5½ or 6 minutes. Then, when you get comfortable with that level, you can increase your daily exercise goal.

✔ **Plan ahead for special activities.** Some activities just take more energy than others, so make special arrangements for them. If you want to go out to lunch with friends, for example, your goal is to have enough energy to keep the date. Resting in the morning, instead of using your energy to clean up the kitchen or straighten the living room, will help you meet this goal.

Establish an Exercise Regimen

Yes, COPD makes you feel short of breath, so you may not think it makes sense to exercise when you already have trouble breathing. But exercise can help you manage your disease and even make breathing easier for you. Regular exercise helps your body use oxygen more efficiently. It helps strengthen your heart, improve your circulation, and lower your blood pressure. And, the more you exercise, the more energy you have, so you feel more like doing the things you like to do.

Your exercise regimen should include stretching, aerobic exercise like walking or riding a stationary bike, muscle toning, and breathing exercises. (Chapter 12 goes into detail about the benefits of exercising with COPD and how to build a regimen that makes sense for you.) When you combine these activities, you strengthen the muscles that help you breathe and move around.

Eat Healthfully

Proper nutrition is just as important as exercise in managing your COPD symptoms. People with COPD burn up to ten times more calories than people without COPD, because they use so much more energy to breathe. Getting enough calories, then, is important, and so is getting the right kind of calories. A healthy diet helps boost your immune system, protecting you against infections like colds and the flu.

A proper diet also is essential for maintaining a healthy weight. Underweight people with COPD are at risk for getting infections, feel weaker and more tired, and generally have greater weakness in the muscles that help them breathe. Being overweight, on the other hand, makes your heart and lungs work harder, makes it harder to get enough oxygen to serve all your body, and can make it harder to breathe by compressing the muscles in your chest and abdomen.

Always talk to your doctor, dietician, or nutritionist before making drastic changes in your diet. However, keep in mind that fruits and vegetables, dairy products, and whole grains all confer specific benefits that can help you manage your COPD and feel better. (See Chapter 11 for more information on how various foods affect your body and your COPD symptoms.)

Use Your Meds Correctly

Your doctor can prescribe all kinds of medications to help open your airways and make breathing easier and more comfortable for you. But if you don't take them properly, they won't help you.

Unfortunately, many COPD patients don't take their medications regularly, and sometimes they even — usually unknowingly — take one medication when they should be taking another. Certainly, the sheer number of prescriptions your doctor hands you can be overwhelming, and the timing of certain medications can be confusing or inconvenient. But skipping doses or taking too much or too little of your medications will not help, and may even hurt, your lung function and overall sense of well-being.

Use these strategies to help you manage your meds correctly and efficiently:

✔ Put your morning, afternoon, and evening meds in separate groups so they don't get mixed up.

✔ To help you remember to take them, put your morning meds next to your toothbrush or the coffeepot — someplace where you'll see them and be reminded to take them every day. Do the same for your other meds.

✔ Use an alarm clock or a wristwatch with an alarm to remind you when it's time to take your timed medications.

✔ Learn how to use your inhalers properly. If you don't know whether you're doing it right, take your inhaler to your next doctor's appointment and ask for help.

Conserve Your Energy

Everybody has high- and low-energy periods throughout the day. When you have COPD, you need to pay attention to your own energy cycle so you can plan activities for times when you'll feel most up to them.

Figuring out ways to save energy is also important. *Remember:* COPD makes you feel tired and weak because you're using so much more energy to breathe. In order to do things *besides* breathe, you may have to figure out ways to make things easier for yourself. This can include

✔ Using a wheeled cart or tray to move things around so you don't have to carry them

✔ Rearranging your routine so you can avoid several trips up and down stairs throughout the day

✔ Scheduling your day so you have rest breaks in between tasks or activities, which gives you a chance to recharge for the next item on your to-do list

Go Easy on Yourself

Don't push yourself to do everything you did when you were 20. Make life easier on yourself by slowing down your pace to help conserve energy. Sit when you can to do tasks like preparing meals, folding laundry, and so on. Choose loose-fitting clothing that won't interfere with breathing, and wear slip-on shoes to avoid bending over.

Pause for a second or two every time you change your body position. When you stand up, wait a moment before beginning to walk; when you get ready to bend over or to straighten up from a bending position, take time to get oriented in your new position before moving again. This simple technique can do much to prevent feeling fatigued or rushed, and when you feel calm, breathing is easier.

Find a Support Group

As awareness of COPD is growing, so too are opportunities to learn from and help support others with the disease. Your doctor's office may be able to refer you to a local support group. You can find lots of resources online, too. Support groups can help you by providing tips and empathy from others who face the same challenges you do. Many people find a great deal of comfort and encouragement in connecting with others who are in the same situation.

Here are some online resources to get you started:

✔ **American Lung Association:** www.lungusa.org

✔ **COPD-Alert:** www.copd-alert.com

✔ **Emphysema Foundation for Our Right to Survive (EFFORTS):** www.emphysema.net

✔ **National Emphysema/COPD Association (NECA):** www.neca community.org

✔ **National Home Oxygen Patients Association:** www.homeoxygen.org

Do Things You Enjoy

One of the reasons COPD patients often suffer from depression is because the disease limits their ability to pursue hobbies and other enjoyable activities, like socializing with friends or going out to museums, or even things like gardening or woodworking.

Accepting your limitations with COPD can be difficult. But finding activities that you can do without overtiring yourself and that will provide you with some enjoyment is important for your mental health — which, incidentally, affects your physical health, too. You may have to get a little creative or delve into your memory to discover or reawaken other interests, but you should consider it an essential part of your COPD therapy.

Look for ways, too, to modify your previous activities so you can still enjoy them. You may not have the energy to go out to dinner every Friday night, but perhaps you can plan ahead for an evening out once or twice a month. If you were accustomed to sewing for an hour every afternoon, maybe you can cut back to half an hour, or plan to sew a couple of times a week instead of every day. Maybe you can play your weekly bingo game online, instead of making the trip to the actual bingo hall.

When it comes to new interests, think about what you always wanted to do when you had time. Maybe you can read the books you never had time for before, for example. Perhaps you always wanted to sketch or do watercolors. Give yourself permission to explore new hobbies, and you may be surprised at how much brighter your mental outlook is, even with COPD.

Let Others Help

Your family and friends are also affected by your COPD. One of the easiest ways to combat their feelings of grief and helplessness is to let them help you with chores and errands.

Don't worry about becoming a burden on your loved ones, or about losing their respect because you don't have the energy to do the things you once did. Family and friends care about you, and they want to be helpful. If you let them do things for you, they'll feel as though they're making a real contribution to your care, and you get to conserve your energy for the things that are really important to you. If letting a family member go to the grocery store or do the laundry for you means you have enough energy to play cards with him this afternoon, everybody feels better.

If you can afford it, consider hiring outside help to come in and do the things you can't or don't want to do any more, like weekly or biweekly housecleaning, mowing the lawn, or shoveling the walks. Hiring someone instead of relying on family and friends to do these things can smooth over the awkwardness that COPD patients and their families sometimes feel: You get to retain some independence without feeling like you're a burden to your loved ones, and your loved ones can relax a bit, knowing that these basic chores are being taken care of.

Chapter 21

Ten (Or So) Health Factors Linked with COPD

A s awareness of and research into COPD gains steam, health professionals are beginning to recognize that COPD actually may be only one *part*
of a broader range of health issues.

In the September 2007 issue of *Lancet,* doctors and pulmonary experts
Leonardo M. Fabbri and Klaus F. Rabe argue that COPD should not be considered simply a lung disease, but a marker for a condition they call *chronic systemic inflammatory syndrome.* They cite the prevalence of other serious
health issues that often coexist with COPD and note that limiting treatment to
COPD symptoms ignores these other factors. COPD rarely shows up without
companions. Many health issues are associated with COPD; some of them
can contribute to development of the disease, and others can be instigated or
made worse by COPD. Here we look at ten of those health issues.

Heart Problems

There's no question that COPD is associated with heart problems: In the
United States, most COPD patients die of heart failure, not respiratory failure,
and one of every five COPD patients also has been diagnosed with chronic
heart failure or congestive heart failure (these two terms are interchangeable).

Like COPD, heart failure is often a long-term disease that gets worse over time, and not just from the effects of aging. High blood pressure, overactive thyroid, previous heart attacks, and several other factors can lead to chronic heart failure. The term *chronic heart failure* means that the heart, little by little, loses its ability to pump efficiently, which may lead to symptoms like shortness of breath and fatigue.

But the exact relationship between COPD and heart problems isn't fully understood. Certainly, when you have COPD, your heart has to work harder to distribute oxygen-rich blood to the rest of your body. And if you're a current or former smoker, your heart (as well as the rest of your body) probably has suffered some inflammatory damage, because smoking attacks not just your lungs but cells throughout your body.

Keep an eye on your ankles. Your ankles may swell occasionally for all kinds of reasons, but if they're consistently swollen, that could be an indication that your heart isn't pumping blood the way it should. When your heart loses its efficiency, blood tends to pool in the lower part of your body, especially in your feet and ankles. If your ankles are regularly swollen, discuss this with your doctor.

Right-heart disease is the most common form of heart trouble in COPD patients, because of the way the circulatory system works: As your blood circulates through your arteries, it distributes oxygen and collects carbon dioxide and other wastes. Then the blood heads back through your veins to the lungs, where it picks up another load of oxygen. The left side of your heart pushes the oxygen-rich blood to your body through your arteries. The blood comes back through your veins to the right side of your heart, which pumps it through your lungs to pick up a new load of oxygen.

Usually, the pressure in the blood vessels and capillaries surrounding your lungs is quite low — only about 20 percent of the blood pressure registered in your arm. But with COPD, your pulmonary blood pressure increases because many of the blood vessels in your lungs are damaged or destroyed, so there are fewer routes to carry the same amount of blood. This increased pressure means the right side of your heart has to work harder to do its pumping. Over time, that extra work can strain and weaken the right heart muscle.

Just having COPD can double or even triple your risk for developing cardiovascular disease, even if you don't smoke and your blood pressure, cholesterol, and weight are all normal. This is another reason exercise is so critical to treating your COPD symptoms: Not only does it help preserve your lung function, but it also helps your heart.

Hardening of the Arteries

Recent research links COPD and *atherosclerosis,* commonly called "hardening of the arteries." This condition increases the risk for heart attacks and strokes because blood flow is restricted or even completely cut off. As COPD gets worse, the walls of the arteries get stiffer, gradually reducing blood flow.

When your lungs are inflamed, they can put pressure on the blood vessels in your chest cavity, including your aorta, the main artery that distributes blood from your heart to the rest of your body. Arteries may respond to this pressure by swelling. After a while, they may "freeze" into a stiff, inflamed state.

The connection between COPD and hardening of the arteries isn't fully understood yet, but inflammation may play a significant role. Both COPD and atherosclerosis are common diseases that are more likely to be found in older people and are linked to smoking, so that may explain why they seem to be related. Nevertheless, there is research that suggests COPD is characterized by *systemic,* or widespread, inflammation, which is known to play a role in making atherosclerosis worse and that, in turn, can lead to damage to the heart.

C-Reactive Protein Levels

C-reactive protein (CRP) is made by the liver, and the liver makes more of it when you have systemic inflammation. Blood tests to measure CRP levels can confirm the presence of systemic inflammation, but they can't pinpoint the location of the inflammation (that is, the blood tests can't determine whether the problem is in your heart, lungs, or knees, to list just three possibilities).

Some research indicates that high CRP levels may predict sudden COPD flare-ups that require hospitalization and even the likelihood of dying from COPD. But not everyone is convinced that this is a reliable indicator because there are other factors besides COPD that can affect CRP production. It's been argued, in fact, that common COPD medications may affect CRP test results.

Elevated levels also are believed to be a primary risk factor for heart disease, but it isn't clear whether high CRP only indicates the presence of heart disease or actually contributes to its development.

Low CRP levels don't necessarily mean there is no inflammation. No one knows why, but people with lupus or rheumatoid arthritis, two diseases that produce chronic inflammation, often have normal CRP test results.

High Blood Pressure

High blood pressure, or *hypertension,* is known as "the silent killer" because, in most cases, people who suffer from it don't have any symptoms. It's quite common, too; an estimated 50 million Americans have it.

When you have COPD, controlling high blood pressure can present some problems. Beta blockers, which are commonly prescribed for hypertension, may not be good for some COPD patients because they interfere with hormones that tell your lungs to open your airways. Fortunately, there are special drugs, called *cardioselective beta blockers,* that focus on the heart and are less likely to be harmful to your airways.

Obesity

Carrying around a few extra pounds doesn't usually affect your lung function — at least not noticeably. But your lung function does decrease as your weight increases, especially your ability to force air out of your lungs. Overweight or obese people who don't have COPD may still feel short of breath because their muscles are forced to work harder to provide normal breathing even when their lungs are normal. That is, their breathing is less efficient. If you can't *exhale* fully, you can't *inhale* fully, either — and that means you can't exchange oxygen for carbon dioxide very well.

Obesity seems to be more commonly associated with chronic bronchitis than with emphysema. The relationship between obesity and COPD is still being studied, but there is some evidence that lack of exercise contributes to COPD as well as obesity.

Weight Loss

For many COPD patients, the problem isn't weight gain but weight loss. Emphysema in particular seems to lead to dangerous loss of muscle tissue, which contributes significantly to the weakness many people with COPD experience. This is why, when you have COPD, eating well (both in terms of nutrition and of quantity) is so important; your body desperately needs the energy that healthy food provides.

Follow these suggestions to make sure you get enough of the right kinds of foods:

- ✔ Eat small meals or snacks five or six times a day instead of larger meals two or three times a day.

- ✔ Keep your kitchen stocked with fresh fruits and vegetables for snacking.

- ✔ Eat soups with vegetables for a snack or light meal.

- ✔ Get most of your protein from sources like poultry and fish instead of beef.

Diabetes

COPD is a risk factor for Type 2 diabetes — also known as non-insulin-dependent, adult-onset, or obesity-related diabetes. As with heart disease, inflammation is believed to be the culprit in making COPD sufferers more susceptible to diabetes. One study indicated that people with COPD are almost twice as likely to develop diabetes as people without COPD.

Although Type 2 diabetes used to be virtually unknown in children and adolescents, its incidence in younger people is rising along with the rise in childhood obesity. The main characteristic of Type 2 diabetes (as opposed to Type 1 diabetes) is that the body, instead of not making enough insulin, becomes resistant to insulin and so requires much higher levels than normal.

Patients with diabetes or glucose intolerance (a pre-diabetes condition) often have problems with blood sugar control when they take medicines like prednisone. Prednisone belongs to a class of drugs called *glucocorticoids,* which are used to treat asthma and severe COPD flare-ups. These drugs cause your liver to release more glucose but prevent your body's tissues from taking in and using sugar from the blood; hence, your blood sugar levels rise.

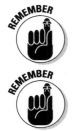

Unless you already have diabetes or glucose intolerance, taking glucocortoids shouldn't present a serious issue.

If you're diabetic and you take certain kinds of steroids to treat severe COPD symptoms, you and your doctor need to monitor your blood sugar levels regularly. When you're hospitalized for severe COPD symptoms, your blood sugar levels should be checked once a day if your diabetes is controlled by diet, every six hours, or before meals and before bed if you're on insulin. At home, you should check your blood sugar before bed and before meals every day if you're taking insulin.

If you have diabetes but are not taking insulin, ask your doctor how often you should check your blood sugar. Most patients check it at least a few times a week; some check it daily. If you're taking steroids for a severe COPD flare-up, your doctor may want you to check your blood sugar more often.

Osteoporosis

Researchers have long known that the kinds of steroid medications often prescribed for COPD can lead to a condition called *drug-induced osteoporosis*. Steroids put your bones at risk because they interfere with your body's ability to absorb and use calcium. When there isn't enough usable calcium circulating in your blood, your body tries to correct the deficiency by breaking down bone materials to release more calcium.

In recent years, though, studies have shown that people with moderate to severe COPD are at higher risk for developing osteoporosis *regardless* of whether they take steroid medications. In the worst cases, people with severe COPD are two and a half times more likely to develop osteoporosis than people with healthy lungs.

If you're taking prednisone or other corticosteroids to treat your COPD symptoms, talk with your doctor about the risks and benefits of your medications. Depending on the severity of your disease and other factors, you may want to try different medications that don't carry as great a risk.

Osteoporosis also can make your COPD symptoms worse, especially if your upper spine has begun to curve into the hallmark hunchback. This severe curving of the spine makes it harder to get air out of and into your chest cavity.

Barrel Chest

When barrel chest comes before you develop COPD, it usually doesn't affect breathing significantly. It's caused by arthritis in the joints that connect your ribs with your spine; the joints calcify, and the ribs get stuck in their expanded, inhaling position. This condition doesn't require treatment and doesn't affect breathing in patients without underlying lung disease.

However, COPD patients sometimes *develop* barrel chest, especially in the late stages of the disease. In this case, the lungs are chronically overinflated, which keeps the ribs pushed out in the inhaling position. It can make breathing even more inefficient and may aggravate the shortness of breath you already feel.

Pulmonary Infections

When you have COPD, not only are you more susceptible to lung infections, but lung infections can be more dangerous, too. This is why we recommend you get a flu shot every year and a pneumonia shot every five years; your immune system needs the boost these vaccines offer.

Children in school or daycare can bring home every bug that's making the rounds in your community. If your grandchildren or other relatives are ill, keep your distance until they're healthy again.

Other lung infections that can cause problems for you include acute bronchitis or pneumonia, which can be caused by bacteria, viruses, or fungi. Even less severe infections can mean a long recovery period when you have COPD.

Call your doctor right away if you have a fever, feel pressure in your chest, are coughing more than normal, or are having a harder time than usual catching your breath. If you're coughing up sputum that is brown, yellow, or green, that could be a sign of infection.

Metabolic Syndrome

Metabolic syndrome is a collection of health issues that includes being overweight, particularly when the concentration of excess weight is carried in the abdomen; resistance to insulin, which can indicate the onset of diabetes; high blood pressure; and low levels of good cholesterol. Sometimes people with metabolic syndrome also have swelling in the legs and feet, which can indicate circulation problems.

About 50 million Americans have metabolic syndrome, which is about four times the number of Americans diagnosed with COPD, and about twice the number of Americans believed to have COPD. It doesn't appear — at least not in the research done so far — that metabolic syndrome is a risk factor for developing COPD. However, people with COPD should be examined for metabolic syndrome to ensure that treatments are appropriate.

Glossary

AAP: *See* alpha antiproteinase (AAP).

AAT: *See* alpha 1-antitrypsin (AAT).

acute: Sudden and usually short-lived. *See also* chronic.

adrenalin: A hormone that causes rapid heartbeat, an increase in blood pressure, and shallow, rapid breathing. Known as the fight-or-flight hormone, adrenalin is released when you sense danger; it also is produced when you smoke.

advance directive: A living will and durable power of attorney for healthcare. These documents provide instructions for your healthcare team and for the person or people you designate to make health treatment decisions for you when you're unable to do so yourself. *See also* durable power of attorney for healthcare *and* living will.

airway: The path air takes to get in and out of your lungs. Your airway includes your nose and mouth, your throat, your trachea (or windpipe), and your bronchi. *See also* trachea *and* bronchi.

airway obstruction: A complete or partial blockage of any portion of the path that air takes to get in and out of your lungs. Allergic reactions, infections, choking, and trauma all can cause airway obstruction.

allergen: Something your body reacts to as if it were dangerous. Common allergens include pollen, mold, and certain foods like peanuts.

allergy: The abnormal response of the airways to allergens in foods or in the air, which can lead to increased mucous production, constriction of the airways, and other symptoms.

alpha antiproteinase (AAP): *See* alpha 1-antitrypsin (AAT).

alpha-1 antitrypsin (AAT): A protein produced by the liver that helps fight inflammation in the lungs. AAT deficiency is a rare genetic defect that almost always leads to emphysema. Also known as alpha antiproteinase (AAP).

alveoli: Tiny sacs at the ends of the smallest airways in the lungs. Their thin walls facilitate the exchange of oxygen and carbon dioxide. One of these sacs is called an *alveolus.*

ambulatory: Able to walk. Your doctor may prescribe *ambulatory oxygen therapy,* which means oxygen you can use while you move around.

antibiotic: A class of medications used to treat infections caused by bacteria. Antibiotics are ineffective against viruses, which is why they are not prescribed for colds and other virus-caused illnesses.

anticholinergic: Medicine that helps open the airways and clear mucus, making coughing more productive. Also called *cholinergic blocker* or *maintenance bronchodilator.*

antihistamine: Medication that blocks histamine receptors in the body, preventing or reducing the severity of symptoms like congestion, sneezing, and watery eyes in response to allergens or cold viruses. *See also* histamine.

anti-inflammatory: Medication that reduces swelling. Common anti-inflammatories include aspirin, ibuprofen, and prednisone, a commonly prescribed steroid.

apnea: Failure to breathe for 10 seconds or longer. Sleep apnea is a common complication of obesity and smoking.

arterial blood gas test: A medical test that measures the amounts of oxygen and carbon dioxide in the blood.

artery: A large blood vessel that carries oxygenated blood throughout your body. The high oxygen content is what makes arterial blood look bright red.

asthma: A lung disorder in which chronic inflammation of the bronchial tubes makes them swell, narrowing the airways. Asthma does not affect air sacs (alveoli).

atelectasis: Collapse of the lung, either partial or complete, usually caused by airways being blocked by fluid or mucus.

bacteria: Single-celled organisms. Some bacteria cause infections in humans and are treated with antibiotics. Also called *germs.*

beta-2 agonist: Medication that relaxes and widens the airways, making breathing easier.

bi-level positive airway pressure (BIPAP): BIPAP machines help you breathe by providing pressure for inhaling and exhaling. *See also* continuous positive airway pressure (CPAP).

BIPAP: *See* bi-level positive airway pressure (BIPAP).

blood pressure: A measurement of the force of blood on the walls of arteries. The higher number is called *systolic* pressure and is measured right after the heart contracts; the lower number is called *diastolic* pressure and is measured right before the heart contracts.

breathing rate: The number of breaths you take per minute. Also called *respiratory rate.*

bronchi: Large tubes that lead from your windpipe to your lungs.

bronchial tubes: Technically, the midsize airways in the lungs that lead to the smallest airways, the bronchioles. In general conversation, *bronchial tubes* may refer to any or all of the airways from your trachea (windpipe) to your lungs. *See also* bronchioles *and* trachea.

bronchioles: The smallest of the air tubes in your lungs. They connect to the air sacs, where oxygen and carbon dioxide are exchanged.

bronchitis: Inflammation and irritation of the bronchial tubes, which causes excessive mucus production and coughing and can lead to difficulty breathing. Bronchitis can be acute or chronic; in COPD, it's chronic.

bronchodilator: A class of medications that help open and clear the airways of mucus. They relax the bands of muscle around the airways to increase airflow. *Fast-acting* bronchodilators are used for acute exacerbations to open airways immediately. *Long-acting* bronchodilators are used to keep airways open and prevent spasms for several hours or longer.

bronchoscopy: A surgical procedure in which a small, lighted camera is passed through the nose or mouth to examine the trachea and bronchi; fluid and tissue also may be removed for further examination or testing.

cannula: A small plastic tube or hose, used to supply oxygen through the nose.

carbon dioxide: A gas that's formed in your body's tissues and expelled through the gas exchange process in your lungs.

carcinogen: Something that causes cancer.

cardiopulmonary resuscitation (CPR): An emergency technique for restoring heartbeat and breathing through chest compression and mouth-to-mouth breathing.

cholinergic blocker: *See* anticholinergic.

chronic: Prolonged, slow to heal, or long-term. *See also* acute.

chronic bronchitis: Long-lasting bronchitis. Your doctor classifies bronchitis as chronic if, for two consecutive years, you have a cough and sputum production every day for at least three months.

cilia: The tiny, hairlike fibers in your lungs that help move mucus and dust up your airways to be coughed out.

closed-mouth technique: *See* open-mouth technique.

compressed oxygen: *See* oxygen, compressed.

continuous positive airway pressure (CPAP): CPAP machines are often prescribed for people with sleep apnea; the machines force open the soft tissues in the throat to facilitate breathing during sleep. *See also* bi-level positive airway pressure (BIPAP).

contraindication: Signs that show a certain treatment or recommendation would not be helpful or would cause further problems. Medicines that are known to interfere with other particular drugs are contraindicated when a patient is already taking those particular drugs.

controlled coughing: A technique that helps clear the airways of mucus but saves energy and oxygen by using only the force needed to loosen and move the mucus. COPD patients learn the controlled coughing technique in pulmonary rehabilitation programs.

cor pulmonale: A condition, common in COPD patients, in which the right side of the heart becomes enlarged in response to elevated pulmonary blood pressure, reducing the heart's efficiency. People with this condition often experience more shortness of breath and swelling in the legs and feet.

corticosteroid: A class of steroid hormones, such as cortisol, made in the cortex, or outer layer, of the adrenal glands. Corticosteroids help reduce inflammation and are often prescribed in either inhaled or tablet form for COPD patients.

CPAP: *See* continuous positive airway pressure (CPAP).

CPR: *See* cardiopulmonary resuscitation (CPR).

cyanosis: The bluish tinge in the skin and mucous membranes that indicates dangerously low levels of oxygen in the blood. In COPD patients, blue-tinted lips or fingernails are indicators of the need for emergency medical attention.

diaphragm: The slightly curved muscle that separates your chest from your abdomen. It drops when you inhale, allowing you to pull air deep into your lungs; when you exhale, it helps force air out of the bottom of your lungs.

diaphragmatic breathing: A technique that allows you to use your diaphragm correctly when breathing, helping you conserve energy. *See also* diaphragm.

dehumidifier: A machine that removes moisture from the air.

dehydration: Severe loss of water from the body.

depression: A diagnosable and treatable illness that affects you physically, mentally, and emotionally. COPD patients may be particularly susceptible to depression when their condition affects their ability to work or take part in activities they enjoy.

diabetes: A chronic illness that involves excessive levels of sugar in the blood and that often is attended by problems with the kidneys, circulatory system, eyes, and other health issues.

diffusion capacity: A measurement of how much oxygen goes from your lungs into your blood.

diuretic: Also known as water pills, diuretics increase your urine output. They're often prescribed for people who have high blood pressure because they help you get rid of excess water. *See also* hypertension.

durable power of attorney for healthcare: A legal document that allows another person, usually a spouse or other family member, to make decisions about your healthcare and treatment when you're unable to make those decisions yourself. *See also* advance directive *and* living will.

dyspnea: Shortness of breath, or difficult or labored breathing.

edema: Swelling, often in the feet or ankles, usually caused by the body's retention of fluid.

emphysema: A lung disease marked by deformation of the air sacs. Air gets trapped in the sacs, stretching them until their natural elastic recoil is lost. The destruction of air sacs makes the gas exchange less efficient. Because air is trapped in the bottom of the lungs, you may feel like you can't get enough air.

environmental tobacco smoke: *See* passive smoking.

exacerbation: A (usually sudden) increase in the severity of symptoms, such as sudden difficulty breathing. Depending on the severity, an acute exacerbation may require a visit to the doctor or even hospitalization.

expectorant: Cough medicine. Expectorants promote productive coughing by thinning out mucus so it can be loosened and coughed out more easily.

exhalation: Forcing air out of the lungs. Also called *expiration.*

expiration: *See* exhalation.

FEV1: *See* forced expiratory volume in the first second (FEV1).

forced expiratory volume in the first second (FEV1): A test to see how well your lungs function. The test measures the volume of air you can force out in 1 second after taking the deepest breath you can.

forced vital capacity (FVC): A test that measures how much air you can force out of your lungs.

FVC: *See* forced vital capacity (FVC).

gas exchange: The process of exchanging oxygen for carbon dioxide in the blood. The gas exchange takes place at the thin walls of the alveoli, where carbon dioxide is taken into the lungs so it can be expelled from the body.

germs: *See* bacteria.

glucose: Sugar. Glucose is the main energy source for living organisms.

heart failure: Failure of the heart to pump blood to meet the body's normal demands, usually because of weakness in the heart muscle. Symptoms of heart failure include swelling in the legs, ankles, or feet, difficulty breathing, and sometimes cyanosis. *See also* cyanosis.

HEPA filter: *See* high-efficiency particulate air (HEPA) filter.

hemoptysis: Bloody sputum or blood coughed up from the lungs. COPD patients who begin coughing up blood or blood-tinged sputum should call for emergency medical help.

high-efficiency particulate air (HEPA) filter: A specially designed filter that removes nearly all tiny particles from the air. People with allergies or COPD often are urged to use HEPA filters in vacuums, furnaces, and air-cleaning devices to reduce the amount of dust in the air.

histamine: A substance that opens blood vessels and makes the vessel walls exceptionally permeable. Histamine plays a major role in allergic reactions; an overabundance of histamine is treated with antihistamines or histamine blockers. *See also* antihistamine.

holding chamber: *See* spacer.

humidifier: A machine that adds moisture to the air.

hypertension: High blood pressure. Your doctor will tell you that you have hypertension if your blood pressure is repeatedly higher than 140/90 (pronounced 140 over 90).

hyperventilation: Overbreathing, which leads to a lower-than-normal level of carbon dioxide in the blood. It can occur because of an increased respiratory rate and/or an increase in the amount of air you move with each breath.

hypoxia: Insufficient oxygen in your body's tissues, even when blood flow is normal.

I/E ratio: The ratio of inhaling to exhaling, or how long you breathe in compared to how long you breathe out.

incentive spirometer: A device that encourages you to breathe as deeply as possible to expand your lungs and help you cough effectively.

inflammation: An immune-system reaction to injury, infection, or other stimuli that includes swelling and sometimes redness.

inhalation: Drawing air into the lungs. Also called *inspiration.*

inhaler: *See* metered dose inhaler (MDI).

inspiration: *See* inhalation.

intubation: A procedure in which a tube is placed in the windpipe to permit artificial breathing.

irritant: Any substance that isn't an allergen but causes you to respond by coughing, sneezing, and so on. Some irritants can damage your lungs. *See also* allergen.

leukotriene modifiers: Medications that reduce the respiratory effects of leukotrienes, which can tighten your airways and promote the production of excessive fluid and mucus.

liquid oxygen: *See* oxygen, liquid.

living will: A legal document that spells out what kind of medical treatment or life-support procedures you want to have or decline if you become unable to make your wishes clear to your family and physician. *See also* advance directive *and* durable power of attorney for healthcare.

lung transplant: A procedure in which a healthy lung from an appropriate donor replaces the recipient's damaged lung.

lung volume reduction surgery: A procedure in which damaged parts of the lung are removed to allow the remaining portion to function better.

maintenance bronchodilator: Generic term for any long-lasting medication (as opposed to rescue medications).

maximal oxygen uptake: Your highest rate of oxygen consumption. This measurement shows your doctor how much oxygen your body uses in one minute.

medical history: An inventory of your previous illnesses, current health and conditions, symptoms, medications (prescribed, over-the-counter, and herbal or supplemental), and risk factors.

metabolism: Your body's use of oxygen and food to create energy. Often expressed as *metabolic rate*. People with a low metabolism generally need fewer calories; those with a higher metabolism need more calories.

metered dose inhaler (MDI): An aerosol canister in a plastic holder that releases a specific amount of medication when you press on the top. The medication comes out in the form of a mist that can be easily inhaled.

mucous: An adjective describing things associated with mucus, such as mucous membranes. *See also* mucus.

mucus: A thick, slick fluid produced by membranes in your mouth, nose, throat, and lungs. Mucus helps keep these body tissues moist and lubricated.

nasal cannula: A small plastic tube with prongs that fit inside the nose, used to deliver oxygen.

nebulizer: A machine that converts liquid medications into a mist that can be easily inhaled through a mask or mouthpiece.

nonsteroidal: An adjective describing medications that aren't steroids. *See also* steroids.

open-mouth technique: The preferred method for inhaling medicine from a metered dose inhaler. The open-mouth technique is more effective than the closed-mouth technique.

orthopnea: Difficulty breathing because of your body position, especially when you experience shortness of breath while lying on your back. Often quantified by the number of pillows needed to relieve the difficulty of breathing.

osteoporosis: Thinning of bones and loss of bone mass because of insufficient calcium and bone protein stores. Osteoporosis raises your risk of fractures that may heal slowly and poorly. Taking steroids for your COPD may increase your risk of developing osteoporosis.

oxygen, compressed: Oxygen that's stored in gas form in a tank under pressure. Flow is controlled through a flow meter and regulator attached to the tank. Compressed oxygen may be prescribed if you only need it for certain activities like walking. Compressed oxygen also is portable, so you can use it when you're away from home.

oxygen, liquid: Liquid oxygen systems store oxygen at very cold temperatures and warm it so it becomes a breathable gas. These systems generally include a large stationary unit and a portable canister that can be filled from the main unit and used when you leave home. The portable canisters typically weigh between 5 and 13 pounds when filled.

oxygen concentrator: A machine that take some air from the room and separates the oxygen from other gases, then delivers the oxygen to you through a nasal cannula. This form of oxygen is most commonly prescribed for people who need to use oxygen while sleeping or who need it 24 hours a day. *See also* nasal cannula.

palpitations: The sensation that your heart is beating unusually rapidly, irregularly, or forcefully. Sometimes palpitations are caused by abnormal heart rhythms; sometimes there is no known cause.

passive smoking: Also called *secondhand smoke* or *environmental tobacco smoke,* passive smoking refers to inhaling smoke from someone else's cigarette — not actively smoking yourself.

peak expiratory flow (PEF) rate: A measurement of how fast you can exhale air from your lungs. Your doctor determines this by using a peak flow meter. (This measurement is generally more applicable when you have asthma than when you have COPD.)

PEF rate: *See* peak expiratory flow (PEF) rate.

phlegm: Mucus. *See also* mucus.

pneumonia: An acute infection of some areas of the lungs that is most commonly caused by bacteria but can also be caused by a virus, a fungus, or a parasite. Symptoms usually include fever, chest pain, productive cough, chills, and difficulty breathing.

postural drainage: A method of positioning your body so gravity helps drain mucus from your lungs.

productive cough: A cough that results in coughing up mucus, which helps you clear your airways.

progressive: In medicine, progressive diseases get worse in increments, becoming more severe and/or affecting more areas of your body. COPD is a progressive disease.

puffer: Common term for *inhaler* or *metered dose inhaler.*

pulmonary: Relating to the lungs.

pulmonary function tests: Tests that measure how well your lungs move air in and out and how efficient they are at getting oxygen into your bloodstream.

pulmonary hypertension: High blood pressure in the arteries in the lungs.

pulmonary rehabilitation: A series of medical treatments, exercises, education, and counseling that helps you learn how to manage your COPD, improve your exercise capacity, and improve your quality of life.

pulmonologist: A physician who specializes in lung disease.

pulse oximetry: A noninvasive test in which a clip on your finger or earlobe measures oxygen levels in your blood. This test can be administered while you're sleeping, sitting still, or exercising. (You may have heard this referred to as a *pulse ox* on your favorite prime-time medical drama.)

pursed-lip breathing: A breathing technique that simulates blowing on a whistle, often recommended for COPD patients to help improve their breathing patterns.

residual volume: How much air is still in your lungs after you breathe out as much as you can.

respiration: The process of breathing in and out.

respiratory failure: The inability of the lungs to perform efficiently and effectively. Respiratory failure can be acute or chronic and is generally defined by low levels of oxygen or high levels of carbon dioxide in the blood.

respiratory rate: *See* breathing rate.

secondhand smoke: *See* passive smoking.

sedentary: Physically inactive, or only slightly active.

side effect: An unpleasant or dangerous response to a medication, usually in addition to the desired effect.

somnolence: Excessive drowsiness or sleepiness. When you have COPD, this can be a sign of dangerously high levels of carbon dioxide in your blood; call for emergency help immediately.

sleep apnea: A disorder in which you stop breathing for 10 seconds or longer at a time during sleep. Your sleep is disrupted because you have to partially wake up to start breathing again; oxygen levels in the blood also may fall perilously low.

spacer: Also called a *holding chamber,* this is a tube that attaches to your metered dose inhaler, making it easier for you to press on the inhaler and breathe in the medicine. *See also* metered dose inhaler (MDI).

spasm: A brief, uncontrollable jerking movement. Muscle spasms and cramps can be caused by nutritional deficiencies like low potassium, by medications, by stress, or by other factors.

spirometry: A test that measures your lungs' air capacity.

steroids: Medications that help reduce swelling and inflammation. COPD patients may be prescribed inhaled steroids or steroids in pill or tablet form.

sputum: Mucus or phlegm. *See also* mucus.

supplement: In nutrition, drinks or tablets that are used to increase your consumption of calories and/or nutrients.

theophylline: A medication that helps open the airways and enhance diaphragmatic function. Not a first-choice medication because of high incidence of side effects and a fairly narrow therapeutic benefit.

tidal volume: How much air you inhale and exhale in one cycle during regular breathing.

total lung capacity test: A test measuring how much air is in your lungs when you've taken as deep a breath as possible.

trachea: Your windpipe, the main airway that supplies both your lungs.

tracheostomy: A surgical procedure in which a small opening is made in the trachea to enable artificial breathing. (The term is commonly used interchangeably with *tracheotomy.*)

tremor: Abnormal, repetitive shaking movement. Tremors can be associated with various diseases and medications; they also can be caused by fever or *hypothermia* (extreme drop in body temperature) and are sometimes related to benign conditions.

vaccine: An injected substance used to prompt your immune system to protect you from specific infections, such as certain strains of flu.

ventilator: The technical term for breathing machines that help support breathing, often used in cases of respiratory failure. Most people use the term *ventilator* to describe the breathing machines hospitals use rather than machines used at home.

virus: An organism, smaller than bacteria, that is highly infectious and contagious. Some 200 viruses are believed to be involved in what we think of as "the common cold," and viruses also are responsible for many other respiratory infections.

vital capacity: How much air you can exhale after you take your deepest possible breath.

wheezing. A high-pitched whistling sound that accompanies breathing when your airways are narrowed by inflammation or scarring.

windpipe: *See* trachea.

withdrawal symptoms: The physical and psychological effects of abruptly discontinuing use of an addictive drug like nicotine. Common withdrawal symptoms include tremors, irritability, anxiety, and inability to sleep.

Index

steroids, 117–119
treatment of acute exacerbations, 259–260
dry cleaning, 243–244
dryers, 226
drying off after bathing, 204
dry-powder inhalers, 124–126
duplicate supplies, 231
durable power of attorney for healthcare, 311
duration, exercise, 195–196
dust
in air as trigger, 283–284
biological, 38
effect on lung function, 30
exposure to, 36
mineral, 35
nuisance, 35
and use of fans, 210
dusting, 229
duties at work, 213
dyspnea, 311

• *E* •

E vitamin, 167
eating. *See also* nutrition
assessing habits, 85
to avoid weight loss, 303
cautions for rest period after, 206
family's understanding of proper habits, 271–272
healthy, as coping strategy, 295
plans, 86
echocardiograms, 84
economic status, 39
edema, 311
EFFORTS (Emphysema Foundation for Our Right to Survive), 269, 297
elasticity, lung, 13, 15, 27
elbow breathing exercises, 191
elbow circles, 191
electric blankets, 212
electric space heaters, 211
emergencies
contacts, 261
emergency plans, 258–261
information to carry in case of, 220

emergency room treatments, 257–258
emotions
attachment to smoking, 157
coping strategies, 74–75
after diagnosis, 64–67
effect of COPD on, 18–19
effect of exercise on, 185–186
finding support, 72–74
managing stress, 70–72
overview, 63–64
role of loved ones in dealing with, 67–70, 266, 274
when disabled, 215
emphysema
damage caused by, 28
defined, 311
overview, 12–13
surgery for, 136–140
Emphysema Foundation for Our Right to Survive (EFFORTS), 269, 297
employers, discussing illness with, 212–213
employment. *See* work
end tables, 225
end-of-life planning
advance healthcare directives, 263–264
desired life-sustaining treatments, 262–263
overview, 261
resuscitation, 263
starting discussion, 261–262
endorphins, 149
endotoxins, 36
endotracheal tubes, 257
energy. *See also* daily life; home
conserving, 296
levels in afternoon, 205–206
loss of, 15–16
mental, 90–91
environment
air quality, 37
dust, 30
pollutants, 30–31
environmental tobacco smoke. *See* secondhand smoke
epiglottises, 22
errands, 218
evenings, 206–207

BUSINESS, CAREERS & PERSONAL FINANCE

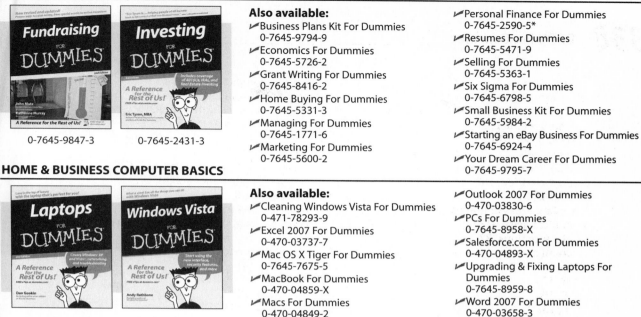

0-7645-9847-3

0-7645-2431-3

Also available:
- Business Plans Kit For Dummies
  0-7645-9794-9
- Economics For Dummies
  0-7645-5726-2
- Grant Writing For Dummies
  0-7645-8416-2
- Home Buying For Dummies
  0-7645-5331-3
- Managing For Dummies
  0-7645-1771-6
- Marketing For Dummies
  0-7645-5600-2

- Personal Finance For Dummies
  0-7645-2590-5*
- Resumes For Dummies
  0-7645-5471-9
- Selling For Dummies
  0-7645-5363-1
- Six Sigma For Dummies
  0-7645-6798-5
- Small Business Kit For Dummies
  0-7645-5984-2
- Starting an eBay Business For Dummies
  0-7645-6924-4
- Your Dream Career For Dummies
  0-7645-9795-7

HOME & BUSINESS COMPUTER BASICS

0-470-05432-8

0-471-75421-8

Also available:
- Cleaning Windows Vista For Dummies
  0-471-78293-9
- Excel 2007 For Dummies
  0-470-03737-7
- Mac OS X Tiger For Dummies
  0-7645-7675-5
- MacBook For Dummies
  0-470-04859-X
- Macs For Dummies
  0-470-04849-2
- Office 2007 For Dummies
  0-470-00923-3

- Outlook 2007 For Dummies
  0-470-03830-6
- PCs For Dummies
  0-7645-8958-X
- Salesforce.com For Dummies
  0-470-04893-X
- Upgrading & Fixing Laptops For Dummies
  0-7645-8959-8
- Word 2007 For Dummies
  0-470-03658-3
- Quicken 2007 For Dummies
  0-470-04600-7

FOOD, HOME, GARDEN, HOBBIES, MUSIC & PETS

0-7645-8404-9

0-7645-9904-6

Also available:
- Candy Making For Dummies
  0-7645-9734-5
- Card Games For Dummies
  0-7645-9910-0
- Crocheting For Dummies
  0-7645-4151-X
- Dog Training For Dummies
  0-7645-8418-9
- Healthy Carb Cookbook For Dummies
  0-7645-8476-6
- Home Maintenance For Dummies
  0-7645-5215-5

- Horses For Dummies
  0-7645-9797-3
- Jewelry Making & Beading For Dummies
  0-7645-2571-9
- Orchids For Dummies
  0-7645-6759-4
- Puppies For Dummies
  0-7645-5255-4
- Rock Guitar For Dummies
  0-7645-5356-9
- Sewing For Dummies
  0-7645-6847-7
- Singing For Dummies
  0-7645-2475-5

INTERNET & DIGITAL MEDIA

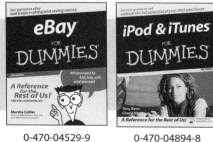

0-470-04529-9

0-470-04894-8

Also available:
- Blogging For Dummies
  0-471-77084-1
- Digital Photography For Dummies
  0-7645-9802-3
- Digital Photography All-in-One Desk Reference For Dummies
  0-470-03743-1
- Digital SLR Cameras and Photography For Dummies
  0-7645-9803-1
- eBay Business All-in-One Desk Reference For Dummies
  0-7645-8438-3
- HDTV For Dummies
  0-470-09673-X

- Home Entertainment PCs For Dummies
  0-470-05523-5
- MySpace For Dummies
  0-470-09529-6
- Search Engine Optimization For Dummies
  0-471-97998-8
- Skype For Dummies
  0-470-04891-3
- The Internet For Dummies
  0-7645-8996-2
- Wiring Your Digital Home For Dummies
  0-471-91830-X

* Separate Canadian edition also available
† Separate U.K. edition also available

Available wherever books are sold. For more information or to order direct: U.S. customers visit www.dummies.com or call 1-877-762-2974. U.K. customers visit www.wileyeurope.com or call 0800 243407. Canadian customers visit www.wiley.ca or call 1-800-567-4797.

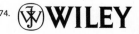

SPORTS, FITNESS, PARENTING, RELIGION & SPIRITUALITY

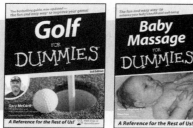

0-471-76871-5

0-7645-7841-3

Also available:

- Catholicism For Dummies
  0-7645-5391-7
- Exercise Balls For Dummies
  0-7645-5623-1
- Fitness For Dummies
  0-7645-7851-0
- Football For Dummies
  0-7645-3936-1
- Judaism For Dummies
  0-7645-5299-6
- Potty Training For Dummies
  0-7645-5417-4
- Buddhism For Dummies
  0-7645-5359-3

- Pregnancy For Dummies
  0-7645-4483-7 †
- Ten Minute Tone-Ups For Dummies
  0-7645-7207-5
- NASCAR For Dummies
  0-7645-7681-X
- Religion For Dummies
  0-7645-5264-3
- Soccer For Dummies
  0-7645-5229-5
- Women in the Bible For Dummies
  0-7645-8475-8

TRAVEL

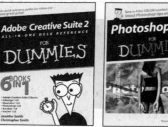

0-7645-7749-2

0-7645-6945-7

Also available:

- Alaska For Dummies
  0-7645-7746-8
- Cruise Vacations For Dummies
  0-7645-6941-4
- England For Dummies
  0-7645-4276-1
- Europe For Dummies
  0-7645-7529-5
- Germany For Dummies
  0-7645-7823-5
- Hawaii For Dummies
  0-7645-7402-7

- Italy For Dummies
  0-7645-7386-1
- Las Vegas For Dummies
  0-7645-7382-9
- London For Dummies
  0-7645-4277-X
- Paris For Dummies
  0-7645-7630-5
- RV Vacations For Dummies
  0-7645-4442-X
- Walt Disney World & Orlando
  For Dummies
  0-7645-9660-8

GRAPHICS, DESIGN & WEB DEVELOPMENT

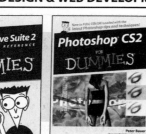

0-7645-8815-X

0-7645-9571-7

Also available:

- 3D Game Animation For Dummies
  0-7645-8789-7
- AutoCAD 2006 For Dummies
  0-7645-8925-3
- Building a Web Site For Dummies
  0-7645-7144-3
- Creating Web Pages For Dummies
  0-470-08030-2
- Creating Web Pages All-in-One Desk
  Reference For Dummies
  0-7645-4345-8
- Dreamweaver 8 For Dummies
  0-7645-9649-7

- InDesign CS2 For Dummies
  0-7645-9572-5
- Macromedia Flash 8 For Dummies
  0-7645-9691-8
- Photoshop CS2 and Digital
  Photography For Dummies
  0-7645-9580-6
- Photoshop Elements 4 For Dummies
  0-471-77483-9
- Syndicating Web Sites with RSS Feeds
  For Dummies
  0-7645-8848-6
- Yahoo! SiteBuilder For Dummies
  0-7645-9800-7

NETWORKING, SECURITY, PROGRAMMING & DATABASES

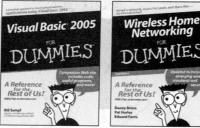

0-7645-7728-X

0-471-74940-0

Also available:

- Access 2007 For Dummies
  0-470-04612-0
- ASP.NET 2 For Dummies
  0-7645-7907-X
- C# 2005 For Dummies
  0-7645-9704-3
- Hacking For Dummies
  0-470-05235-X
- Hacking Wireless Networks
  For Dummies
  0-7645-9730-2
- Java For Dummies
  0-470-08716-1

- Microsoft SQL Server 2005 For Dummies
  0-7645-7755-7
- Networking All-in-One Desk Reference
  For Dummies
  0-7645-9939-9
- Preventing Identity Theft For Dummies
  0-7645-7336-5
- Telecom For Dummies
  0-471-77085-X
- Visual Studio 2005 All-in-One Desk
  Reference For Dummies
  0-7645-9775-2
- XML For Dummies
  0-7645-8845-1

HEALTH & SELF-HELP

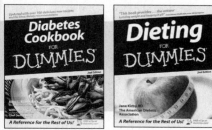

0-7645-8450-2   0-7645-4149-8

Also available:
- Bipolar Disorder For Dummies
  0-7645-8451-0
- Chemotherapy and Radiation For Dummies
  0-7645-7832-4
- Controlling Cholesterol For Dummies
  0-7645-5440-9
- Diabetes For Dummies
  0-7645-6820-5* †
- Divorce For Dummies
  0-7645-8417-0 †

- Fibromyalgia For Dummies
  0-7645-5441-7
- Low-Calorie Dieting For Dummies
  0-7645-9905-4
- Meditation For Dummies
  0-471-77774-9
- Osteoporosis For Dummies
  0-7645-7621-6
- Overcoming Anxiety For Dummies
  0-7645-5447-6
- Reiki For Dummies
  0-7645-9907-0
- Stress Management For Dummies
  0-7645-5144-2

EDUCATION, HISTORY, REFERENCE & TEST PREPARATION

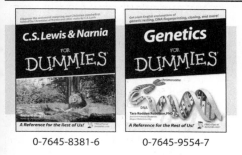

0-7645-8381-6   0-7645-9554-7

Also available:
- The ACT For Dummies
  0-7645-9652-7
- Algebra For Dummies
  0-7645-5325-9
- Algebra Workbook For Dummies
  0-7645-8467-7
- Astronomy For Dummies
  0-7645-8465-0
- Calculus For Dummies
  0-7645-2498-4
- Chemistry For Dummies
  0-7645-5430-1
- Forensics For Dummies
  0-7645-5580-4

- Freemasons For Dummies
  0-7645-9796-5
- French For Dummies
  0-7645-5193-0
- Geometry For Dummies
  0-7645-5324-0
- Organic Chemistry I For Dummies
  0-7645-6902-3
- The SAT I For Dummies
  0-7645-7193-1
- Spanish For Dummies
  0-7645-5194-9
- Statistics For Dummies
  0-7645-5423-9

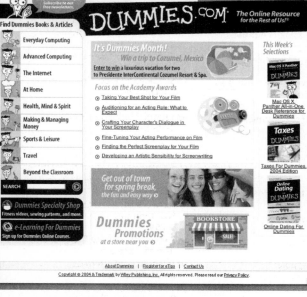

Get smart @ dummies.com®

- **Find a full list of Dummies titles**
- **Look into loads of FREE on-site articles**
- **Sign up for FREE eTips e-mailed to you weekly**
- **See what other products carry the Dummies name**
- **Shop directly from the Dummies bookstore**
- **Enter to win new prizes every month!**

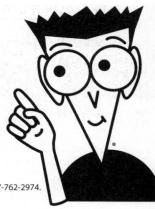

* Separate Canadian edition also available
† Separate U.K. edition also available

Available wherever books are sold. For more information or to order direct: U.S. customers visit www.dummies.com or call 1-877-762-2974.
U.K. customers visit www.wileyeurope.com or call 0800 243407. Canadian customers visit www.wiley.ca or call 1-800-567-4797.

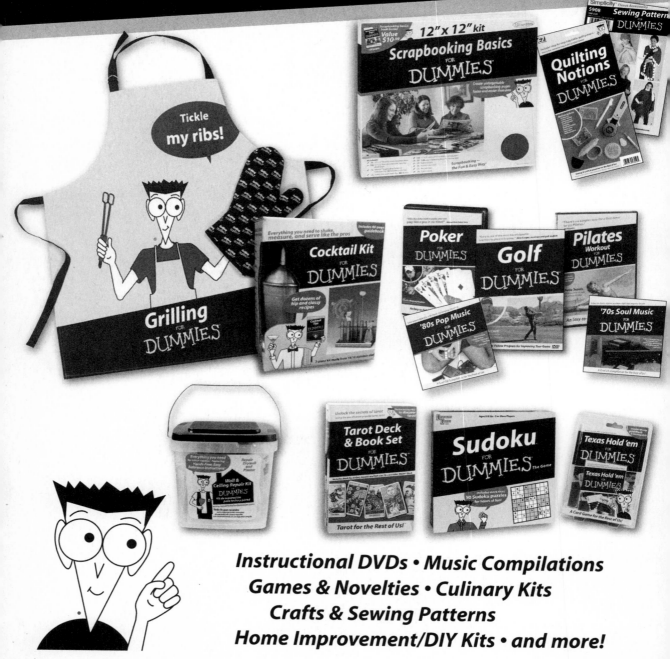
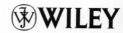